Vet Confidential

Vet
Confidential

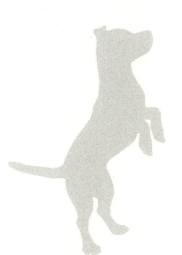

AN INSIDER'S GUIDE
TO PROTECTING YOUR
PET'S HEALTH

Louise Murray, D.V.M.

Ballantine Books   New York

> *To my own beautiful family—Peter, Dov, and Siena—and to all*
> *the other families made up of both two- and four-legged beings*

The material in this book is supplied for informational purposes only and is not meant to take the place of a veterinarian's advice. No book can replace the diagnostic expertise and medical advice of a trusted professional. Please be certain to consult with your vet before making any decisions that affect your pet's health, particularly if they suffer from any medical condition or have any symptom that may require treatment. Similarly, while there is information in the book concerning laws and regulations relevant to veterinary care, this area is complex and constantly changing. You should, therefore, consult with an experienced attorney to apply the relevant laws in your state to your unique situation.

Copyright © 2008 by Louise Murray, D.V.M.

All rights reserved.

Published in the United States by Ballantine Books, an imprint of The Random House Publishing Group, a division of Random House, Inc., New York.

BALLANTINE and colophon are registered trademarks of Random House, Inc.

As of press time, the URLs displayed in this book link or refer to existing websites on the Internet. Random House, Inc., is not responsible for the content available on any such site (including, without limitation, outdated, inaccurate, or incomplete information).

Library of Congress Cataloging-in-Publication Data

Murray, Louise.
  Vet confidential : an insider's guide to protecting your pet's health
/ Louise Murray.
      p. cm.
Includes bibliographical references and index.
ISBN 978-0-345-50320-6 (hardcover : alk. paper)
1. Pets—Health.   2. Pets—Diseases.   3. Veterinary medicine.   I. Title.

SF413.M78 2008
636.089—dc22
2008005064

Printed in the United States of America on acid-free paper

www.ballantinebooks.com

9 8 7 6 5 4 3 2 1

First Edition

Book design by Nancy B. Field

CONTENTS

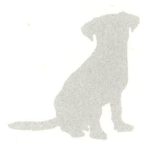

YOU Can Help Your Pet
Mehmet C. Oz, M.D.

My family currently shares our home with five cats, three hamsters, two angelfish, a rabbit, and a box turtle. The only thing we're missing is a partridge in a pear tree. My wife and kids feel that my work as a cardiothoracic surgeon should give me deep insight when one of our cats is limping or a hamster has a runny nose, but the real truth is that when it comes to our animals, I need the help of a good vet—just like you do. Needless to say, with all these beloved critters in the house, veterinary medicine plays a continuous and valuable role in our lives. It's important to us that our menagerie has the best medical care, and we're always on the lookout for ways to keep everyone healthy and happy. We also feel that the kids learn compassion and responsibility through the experience.

As a physician and an author, I always emphasize that the most important step you can take for your own health is to really understand how your body works. By taking your health into your own hands—for example, learning why diseases occur, and what causes aging—you can live longer, and look and feel your very best. Knowing your body gives you the motivation to keep it young and strong.

The same concepts hold true concerning the well-being of our pets. Just as we can control our own health destinies through knowledge, we can protect our pets by learning as much as we can. Yet reliable advice isn't always easy to come by, regarding our own health or that of our animals. With all the news stories, scientific reports, and medical recommendations that bombard us, it can seem virtually impossible to reach into the constant stream of data and grasp the most important facts. When we wrote *YOU: The Owner's Manual,* our goal was to haul out the best catch of useful information from that stream and present it in a way that was easy to comprehend, and hopefully fun as well.

In *Vet Confidential,* Dr. Murray does the veterinary fishing for you, netting the essentials from a sea of confusing and sometimes contradictory information and delivering them to you in a clear and concise fashion. She also dishes out some facts you probably won't find anywhere else. By the way, did you know that high blood pressure is as dangerous for pets as it is for us, or that veterinary ophthalmologists can perform cataract surgery similar to that done for humans? Maybe this is the first time you've heard that there is even such a thing as a veterinary ophthalmologist! *Vet Confidential* takes you inside veterinary medicine, so you can become an educated partner in your pet's medical care. What you learn may amaze you, and will certainly help you keep your pet happy and well.

If you've read any of my books, you know that I'm a big fan of quizzes. Here are five questions on topics that are essential for your pet's well-being. Take a few moments to see how you do.

The Pet Health Quiz:
How Much Do You Know About Veterinary Medicine?

1. Every dog should be vaccinated against _____.
    a. The intestinal parasite *Giardia*.
    b. Canine parvovirus.
    c. Rattlesnake venom.
    d. Lyme disease.

2. Every cat should be vaccinated against _____.
    a. The feline leukemia virus.
    b. Feline immunodeficiency virus.
    c. Feline coronavirus.
    d. Feline panleukopenia virus.

3. If the veterinarian hears a heart murmur during your cat's physical exam, the safest plan would be to:
    a. Have a chest X-ray taken; if it's normal, there's nothing to worry about.
    b. Have the murmur monitored yearly to make sure it doesn't get any louder.
    c. Have a cardiac ultrasound performed by a veterinary cardiologist.
    d. Put your cat on a low-fat diet.

4. Which of the following is *not* true regarding high blood pressure in pets?
    a. High blood pressure is common in older pets, especially those with certain health conditions.
    b. Untreated high blood pressure can result in sudden blindness in cats and dogs.
    c. It is difficult to measure blood pressure in pets, especially those weighing less than ten pounds.
    d. Some of the same medications used to treat high blood pressure in people are also used for this purpose in dogs and cats.

5. You move to a different city and you're looking for a new veterinary practice. It's most important to choose a veterinary practice that _____.
    a. Is as close to your house as possible so your pet won't have to travel too far.
    b. Uses up-to-date monitoring equipment on animals under anesthesia.
    c. Has a large waiting room with separate areas for dogs and cats.
    d. All your new neighbors use.

Answers to the Pet Health Quiz

1. b. Canine vaccines are considered to fall into three categories: core vaccines, which every dog should receive; noncore optional vaccines, which are used in certain dogs based on geographic location and lifestyle; and vaccines that are not generally recommended. Because canine parvovirus is widespread and highly infectious, it is recommended that all dogs be vaccinated against this disease.

2. d. Feline vaccines are also categorized as core, noncore optional, and not generally recommended. On this list, only feline panleukopenia is considered a core vaccine, and all cats should be vaccinated against this devastating infection.

3. c. While chest X-rays are useful in cats with heart murmurs, only a cardiac ultrasound can be used to accurately diagnose a cat with heart disease and ascertain whether medication is necessary. It is not possible to tell whether a cat has significant heart disease by listening to a heart murmur—in fact, some cats with heart disease don't have a murmur at all. Low-fat diets are not used for cats with heart disease.

4. c. Blood pressure can easily be measured in dogs and cats. High blood pressure occurs in many middle-aged and older pets, particularly those with kidney disease or hormonal conditions. Severely elevated blood pressure that is not discovered and treated can cause blindness due to retinal damage.

5. b. Although your pet may not enjoy traveling to the veterinarian, it is much more essential for your pet's safety that you use a practice that will properly monitor your pet during anesthesia.

Odds are you just realized that you didn't learn everything you needed to know about veterinary medicine in the pet store. Now is your chance to get your honorary doctorate. Just as it is true for your own health, the more you know, the better care you can take of your pet—so here's to a long and healthy life for both of you!

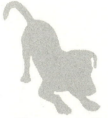

Standards of Care:

The Informed Veterinary Consumer

Let's face it: We are a nation of pet lovers. There are more than ninety million pet owners in the United States, and about 160 million pet dogs and cats (yep, they outnumber us!). To many of us, our pets are like family members . . . in fact, they *are* family members, albeit rather furry ones. Gone are the days when Rover was relegated to the doghouse out back and Fluffy got a bowl of milk once in a while if she was lucky. Now our pets sleep where we sleep, eat what we eat, and often travel wherever we go, too (in fact, these days room service has a menu just for them).

I look around me and smile at the evidence. I walk to work past doggy day care centers and canine play groups in the park. I see shoppers carefully selecting among myriad brands and flavors of cat food, staring at labels, and offering advice to one another: "Freddy loves their Trout Terrine, but he wouldn't even *touch* the Salmon Soufflé." Our pets have salons, spas, and sitters, designer coats and collars, food so gourmet you could serve it at your next cocktail party, and cookbooks with recipes just for them. Even their names have changed; instead of Spot and Tabby, veterinary practices now care for William, Lucy, Megan, and Matthew.

We're always on the lookout for the best products for our pets—the most wholesome food, the safest toys, the comfiest carriers. We want to protect our pets and make sure that they live long, happy lives. Yet more important than any product we could purchase is their health care. It's easy to pick out the most stylish collar for your pet, but how do you choose the right veterinarian? How do you know if your pet is receiving proper medical treatment or the most effective therapy when she's sick?

For our own health, there are expected standards of practice. The human medical profession is held to stringent criteria, and patients and their families are vigilant in judging the care they have received. People are adept at finding the right doctor or specialist: requesting referrals, searching medical directories for recommendations, or canvassing friends and colleagues. We painstakingly research symptoms and illnesses on medical websites. We expect to be fully informed by our doctors and don't hesitate to seek a second opinion when we have doubts. Pet owners should be equally demanding consumers. You should be able to rely on certain standards of care from the veterinary profession and have the resources to help you ensure this is the case.

Veterinary medicine has made remarkable progress. Yet there is still much disparity in the health care provided for pets. As a practicing veterinarian, blessed to have met so many devoted pet owners, I've discovered that most are unaware of the standard of veterinary care they should expect for their pets or the current developments in the field that could benefit their animals. Often, they learn too late to help a pet in need. Not only should pet owners be able to expect a high standard of general health care, but they should also be given the opportunity to take advantage of the latest advances when a pet's health requires it. The days are past when there was only one vet in town and little that could be done for a sick animal. Now pet owners have choices, and they deserve the knowledge that will allow them to make best use of those choices for their pets' well-being.

My goal is to give you that knowledge. Whether you're choosing a general veterinarian or seeking help for an animal who has become ill, you should have the tools to ensure that your pet receives the best care possible. Our canine and feline companions have become very important to us, and the public is now questioning the veterinary profession, from the vaccines we use to the drugs we prescribe. Many pet owners feel lost when their pets become ill—unsure where to turn or who to trust. When these issues arise, people may look to unreliable sources of information on the Internet or elsewhere. This book will help you to become informed so that you can pick the right veterinary practice for your pet, demand the best treatment if he becomes ill, and protect yourself from dubious advice from any source.

By becoming an informed veterinary consumer, you won't just benefit your own pet; you'll be protecting *all* of them. How? By helping to raise the bar for every pet's health care. If pet owners begin selecting veterinary practices that can measure pets' blood pressure, maybe one day every practice will have this equipment. If enough pet owners insist that their pets be properly monitored while under anesthesia, someday every pet will have this safeguard. If more pet owners request pain medication for a pet who has had surgery, maybe it will be prescribed for others as well. If owners of sick pets inquire about referral to a specialist, perhaps this option will be suggested more often.

Veterinary medicine is an amazing profession. I see in it the best side of human nature; surely giving care to those of another species is a manifestation of the goodness that is in us. Whenever I begin to take this for granted, a moment will come when I step back and suddenly glimpse again how remarkable it truly is. And the bond between pets and their human guardians is a similarly wonderful thing: a love that crosses species boundaries and brings warmth and happiness to the lives of so many. Our job as veterinarians is to safeguard that bond by doing our utmost to keep pets healthy and safe, and being a trustworthy resource for pet owners to rely on. We have a responsibility to live up to the faith that is placed in us.

A word about language: Many people are no longer comfortable with the phrase *pet owner*, protesting that our pets are not property as this term implies. In fact, some would do away with the word *pet* as well, feeling that it diminishes the essential role animals play in our lives, as family members, friends, and valued companions. Yet no satisfactory replacements are currently in place for this terminology. In my profession, we often refer to people as their pets' parents; it is common for a veterinarian to say, "Phoebe's dad called to say she's been vomiting again," or "Max's mom is coming to pick him up at six."

However, there are those who are not quite ready to be referred to as the parents of their dogs and cats. *Human guardian* has been proposed but is rather awkward; *animal companion* has been substituted for *pet* but is also fairly cumbersome. So, with apologies, I have chosen to stick with *pet* and *pet owner* for now, due to the lack of ready alternatives. These terms have not seemed to hinder the relationship between my patients and their people, so I can live with them for the time being, and hopefully you will forgive their use in this book.

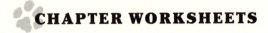

CHAPTER WORKSHEETS

At the end of each chapter, you will find one or more relevant worksheets. These have been designed to help you put the information in this book to practical use for your own pet. Some provide summaries of relevant points that were covered so that you have the most important facts readily at hand; others are checklists that you can use as aids in various aspects of your pet's health care. The aim of this book is to help you to become a knowledgeable and effective advocate for your pet's health, working in partnership with a trusted veterinarian to keep your furry family members vital and happy. I hope these worksheets will make it a bit easier for you to achieve that goal.

Vet Confidential

CHAPTER 1

On the Scent:

Tracking Down the Best Veterinary Practice for Your Pet

You've decided to become an informed veterinary consumer, and this decision is going to greatly benefit your pet's well-being. The first step toward your goal of ensuring that your pet receives the very best health care available is to carefully select a veterinarian. Just as in every profession, there can be real differences among veterinary practices. By learning what to look for (and what to avoid), you will be able to make educated decisions with your pet's particular needs in mind. There are many excellent practices providing up-to-date, high-quality medicine, and others that are unable to offer the same level of care or have fallen behind. The key for pet owners is to possess the tools to make an accurate assessment and choose wisely.

How do I choose the right veterinarian for my pet?

There are various times when you need to select a veterinarian. Maybe you've just brought home a new pet (or two). Or perhaps you've recently moved and are searching for a good practice nearby. If your pet has developed health problems, you may suddenly find it more important than ever that she has the best care available. You may even have concerns about your current veterinary practice and be considering a change.

When you find yourself looking for a veterinarian—for whatever reason—what's the best way to go about choosing the right one for your pet?

If you're like most people, you have some personal preferences that may influence your choice. Maybe there's a practice that's in a particularly convenient location or has hours best suited to your schedule. Perhaps you feel your dog is more comfortable with a female doctor, or your cat is happier in practices that handle only felines. There may be a local veterinary hospital that your family has trusted for years, or that a friend recommends.

These considerations are indeed important, but you should also weigh some objective criteria when deciding which doctor to entrust with your pet's well-being. If you have a choice of practices in your area, you want to use the one that offers your pet the highest standard of care and avoid those that aren't achieving the quality of medicine you're seeking. To help you in your search, I've compiled a list of questions that will enable you to evaluate various aspects of each veterinary practice you consider. The areas covered include patient care, equipment, staffing, philosophy, and how up-to-date the facility is. Using this checklist, you will gain the ability to more knowledgeably oversee your pet's health care.

🐾 THE CHECKLIST

The checklist is divided into two sections. The first contains questions about the veterinary practice you're considering that can be answered over the phone by a staff member. The second section contains topics that are best evaluated during an appointment. There are two worksheets at the end of the chapter where you can record the information you gather.

One option when you're evaluating a new practice is to schedule an appointment to take place without your pet. This will allow you and the veterinarian to focus on your concerns and have enough time for an informative discussion. Also, since your pet won't have been seen at the practice, you may feel less awkward if you decide not to return. Be prepared to pay the normal fee for the appointment, even though your pet is not present. Don't feel hesitant about letting the veterinarian know that you are trying to pick the right practice for your pet; many parents interview several pediatricians before selecting a doctor for their children, and you, too, have every right to do some investigating.

If this suggestion is not convenient or affordable for you, you can evaluate the practice during your pet's first visit. You probably shouldn't expect to be able to stop by a practice your pet has never been to and speak to the veterinarian without an appointment.

What if I am too shy to ask these kinds of questions?

We all sometimes find ourselves losing our voice: at the doctor's or veterinarian's office or even the hair salon. We don't want to annoy or impose upon anyone, and we feel embarrassed to speak up. Keep in mind that veterinary practices are there to serve you and your pet. You are entrusting them with your pet's well-being, and you are paying for their services. You certainly wouldn't buy a car or choose a vacation spot without asking plenty of questions and having a sense of what to expect. I bet you feel more strongly about your pet's health than either of those. So ask away!

I appreciate clients who care enough to ask questions; they allow me to practice the best medicine. Always remember that a veterinarian should value a client like you and be gracious in addressing your concerns. If not, you may want to consider another practice.

What if I have concerns about my pet's current veterinary practice?

You can use the checklist to help you evaluate your current veterinary practice and perhaps pinpoint the cause for your concern. I'm surprised by how many pet owners stay with a practice despite being uncomfortable there or dissatisfied with their pet's care. They may not realize that there can be significant differences among practices, or they may feel awkward about leaving, particularly if they are long-term clients. The truth is that veterinarians are accustomed to clients coming and going. As professionals, they see this as a normal part of doing business. Like any other relationship, there must be a good fit between you and your veterinarian; if it doesn't feel right, it is perfectly natural to consider a change. Your pet's health must always be your top priority. Your decisions should be made with that responsibility in mind.

Sometimes people are unsure about how to diplomatically go about shifting their pet's care from one veterinarian to another. If you decide to try a different practice, simply ask that a copy of your pet's complete records be mailed to you. You don't need to indicate the reason why you want the file, or that you have decided to take your pet elsewhere.

How can I narrow down the practices in my area?

You can start by finding out which practices are accredited by the American Animal Hospital Association (AAHA). Participation is voluntary, and whether or not a practice has chosen to be evaluated by the AAHA can be an indication of its commitment to providing a high level of care. AAHA accreditation involves an on-site evaluation to determine if the practice meets all the standards established by the association, and then periodic reviews to ensure that it continues to meet those standards. The practice is graded in many areas, including the facility, staff, equipment, and patient care. Only veterinary hospitals that meet the rigorous AAHA standards receive accreditation.

You can look for accredited practices on the AAHA's website (www.healthypet.com) or in the phone book, or by calling local practices to inquire about their status.

TIP Another good way to find a practice in your area is to get a recommendation from an equally concerned pet owner. Ask your friends, neighbors, and colleagues for the name of their veterinarian and how they feel about the practice. But be sure to ask specific questions, such as the ones that follow. It's wonderful that your neighbor loves her dog's doctor, but you need to make sure the practice provides the level of care you are looking for.

CHECKLIST: BEFORE YOU MAKE AN APPOINTMENT

To see if a practice meets your needs, you can ask the following preliminary questions over the telephone. A staff member should be cheerfully willing and able to give you this information. If the person who answers the phone can't supply all the answers, ask to speak to the office manager or medical director. Explain that you are looking for a veterinarian for your pet and that you would like to learn more about their practice. It is perfectly acceptable for them to request to return your call if they are busy.

1. How are patients in the hospital monitored during the night?

If your pet should ever require overnight hospitalization, you must be confident that he will receive adequate care. Some pets are hospitalized primarily for the purpose of cage rest—for example, an animal with a bandage, splint, or fracture who may suffer further injury from too much movement. In situations such as this, the pet doesn't necessarily need to be observed during the night.

A pet who is ill or recovering from surgery, however, can benefit greatly from being monitored overnight. For example, the animal will be able to receive necessary medications and intravenous fluids throughout the night. Patients who are on IV fluids should receive them continuously, and this must be closely supervised. And if something serious happens, such as bleeding, severe discomfort, or deterioration of the animal's condition, overnight monitoring can prove crucial and sometimes lifesaving.

The degree of overnight care provided varies widely among veterinary practices. Some practices are unable to provide any type of care at night; some have an employee who intermittently stops by to check on the patients or administer treatments. Other practices have one or more veterinary technicians and/or doctors treating and monitoring the patients throughout the night.

A practice that does not provide overnight care may suggest that your pet be hospitalized at another facility until she is more stable. Some practices have an arrangement whereby the animals are transferred to an overnight care facility during the night, and then returned to the practice during the day. This can be cumbersome for owners, who are generally the ones transporting their pets back and forth, but it does provide a safety net. In any case, the situation you want to avoid is one in which your pet is left alone overnight when doing so may threaten her health or comfort.

Many excellent veterinarians practice in situations where the cost of having an overnight employee is not warranted. Naturally, some smaller practices are not as equipped as larger animal hospitals to deal with very ill or postoperative patients. What matters is that the practice handles these situations appropriately by referring patients to another facility when needed. It's crucial that the practice recognizes that the need for overnight care can arise, and that they have established a plan ensuring that such care is provided when necessary for the patient's safety, whether at their office or at another facility. Avoid using a practice where sick or postoperative patients are kept alone at night.

Questions to ask:

- How do you handle overnight care for your patients?
- Is there an overnight employee? If so, is she monitoring the patients continuously, or does she stop by periodically?
- Is the overnight employee either a veterinarian or licensed veterinary technician?

---

2. Does the practice use adequate and modern equipment?

Veterinary practices vary widely in their equipment. Still, certain types of equipment are so essential, I recommend you select a practice that has them on the premises. These four examples can be used as benchmarks to help assess whether the practice is well equipped and up-to-date.

Blood pressure equipment: Just like in people, many health conditions cause animals to develop perilously high or low blood pressure, and this relatively simple equipment can make an enormous difference in your pet's care. For example, animals can have high blood pressure that leads to a stroke or blindness (especially those with kidney disease or hormonal disorders), and animals who are under anesthesia or very ill may develop dangerously low blood pressure. You might be surprised to learn how many veterinary practices do not have this basic item and cannot measure their patients' blood pressure.

PCV centrifuge: A PCV centrifuge allows veterinarians to quickly measure an animal's red blood cell level using a small blood sample called a PCV, or packed cell volume. This equipment can be lifesaving for patients who are anemic or have blood loss. For example, during surgery, an animal may lose enough blood to require a transfusion. With a PCV centrifuge, the patient's red blood cell level can be measured immediately, instead of waiting for a blood test to be sent out to a laboratory. Without this equipment, it is difficult for a practice to safely handle such situations.

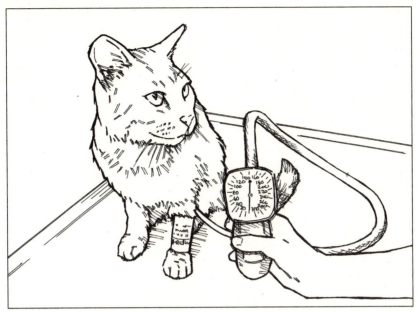

A cat having his blood pressure measured with a cuff on the front leg

Pulse oximeter: A pulse oximeter is used to monitor an animal's oxygen level. This is critical for patients under anesthesia as well as for those who have difficulty breathing, such as pets with pneumonia or heart failure.

Radiology equipment: Most veterinary practices have radiology equipment, but not all of the equipment will be of the same quality. For example, older machines require the X-rays to be developed by hand; newer automatic processors for film development result in higher-quality diagnostic radiographs. Poor-quality radiographs are much harder to interpret, and important information can be missed. The latest technology in this area is digital radiography, which is more commonly found in very large or specialized practices. I recommend you choose a practice that uses an automatic processor—or has digital radiography, which does not require developing.

If possible, choose a practice that has all these pieces of equipment. If this is not available in your area, choose the one that seems best equipped or best meets all the other standards.

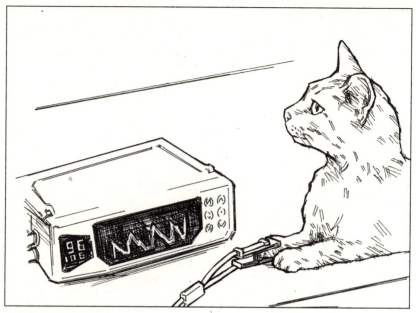

A cat having his blood oxygen level measured with a pulse oximeter on his paw

---

Questions to ask:

- Do you have equipment to measure patients' blood pressure?

- Do you have equipment to measure patients' red blood cell levels, such as a PCV centrifuge?

- Do you have equipment to measure patients' oxygen levels, such as a pulse oximeter?

- Do you use an automatic processor to develop X-rays? (Or do you have digital radiography?)

---

3. Does the practice refer patients to specialists?

There are many veterinary specialties, and at some point referral to a specialist or advanced care facility may be necessary for your pet. I'll be discussing this in much more detail in chapter 4. For example, an animal who needs major surgery may be referred to a surgeon, one with a heart murmur may be referred to a cardiologist, and one with liver disease, kidney failure, or another organ problem may be referred to an internist.

Besides offering expertise in particular areas of medicine, specialty practice groups also provide a heightened level of care. For example, an animal who is very sick or in need of major surgery may be referred to a facility with an intensive care unit (ICU) featuring advanced monitoring capabilities and nursing around the clock.

You want to be sure that your chosen veterinary practice is willing to refer your pet, when it's in his best interest, to a specialist or advanced care facility. Think of it this way: Referring a patient to a specialist is like passing the ball to someone who is in a better scoring position—an unselfish act for the greater good. You don't want to be on a team with someone who hogs the ball.

You should be concerned if the practice's approach is *We don't need to refer, we can do everything here,* especially if the practice does not offer a variety of board-certified specialists as well as twenty-four-hour care. This philosophy should make you concerned about your pet's safety as well as the practice's priorities.

Questions to ask:

- Do you refer critical patients to an advanced care facility? If so, which one?
- In what situations do you refer patients to a specialist?
- Do you refer patients to specialists for major surgery or advanced diagnostic procedures such as ultrasound?
- Do you refer patients who have conditions that are difficult to diagnose or treat to specialists for a second opinion?

---

4. Are modern anesthetic techniques employed?

I cannot stress strongly enough how important this issue is for your pet. When evaluating whether a practice is using the safest and most current methods of anesthesia, there are three critical factors to look for.

First, find out the type of anesthesia that is used by the practice. The current standard of care is that patients undergoing surgery are anesthetized using one of the modern types of gas anesthesia. Only very brief procedures such as replacing a splint or taking an X-ray should be performed under injectable sedation.

TIP The two modern types of gas anesthesia commonly used by veterinarians are *isoflurane* and *sevoflurane. Halothane,* an older gas anesthetic, is not as safe. Do not use a practice that performs surgery without using modern gas anesthesia.

Second, any patient under anesthesia should have an IV catheter in place. During an anesthetic emergency, the catheter is used to quickly deliver potentially lifesaving drugs and fluids. For example, if an animal's heart rate becomes dangerously low, a drug called atropine can be injected; if her heart stops, a drug called epinephrine can be given; and if her blood pressure drops too low, intravenous fluids and drugs can be delivered to correct this.

Third, patients should be intubated while under anesthesia. Intubation, which is the placement of a tube in the trachea (windpipe), greatly increases the safety of a patient under anesthesia. The tube delivers oxygen to the patient to keep levels adequate, and if his breathing slows or stops, or his oxygen level drops too low, the tube can be used to assist the animal in breathing. During respiratory or cardiac arrest, the tube can be used for

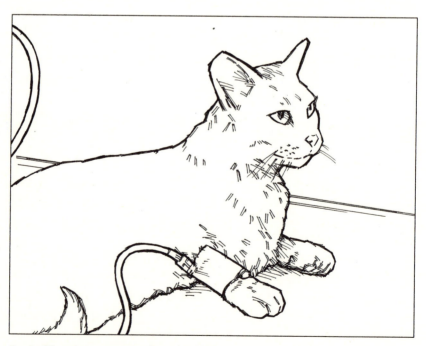

A cat with an intravenous catheter in place

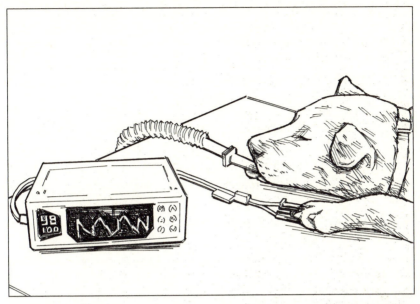

A tube has been placed in the trachea of this anesthetized dog to safely administer anesthetic gas and oxygen, and to prevent saliva or regurgitated food from entering the lungs. The dog has a pulse oximeter on his paw to monitor his blood oxygen level.

prompt resuscitation. In addition, while the animal is anesthetized and unable to swallow or cough on his own, the tube prevents saliva, blood, or regurgitated food from entering the trachea and lungs.

Questions to ask:

- What types of modern gas anesthetics are used at the practice?
- Do patients have an intravenous catheter placed prior to anesthetic procedures?
- Are patients intubated during anesthesia?

5. Are patients properly monitored during anesthesia?

With current technology, there are many ways to monitor a patient under anesthesia. The oxygen level, heart rhythm, and blood pressure can be measured continuously. This type of monitoring is crucial in preventing anesthetic fatalities; by warning the doctor and technician that the patient's oxygen level or heart rate is falling, it allows intervention to occur before it is too late.

Ideally, the practice should use equipment that allows all three of these vital signs to be followed during anesthesia. At a minimum, the pet's oxygen level and pulse rate should be monitored during the procedure by a pulse oximeter, which displays the blood oxygen level and heart rate continuously. If your pet has had anesthesia, you can ask to see her medical file, where there should be a record of her vital signs noted throughout the time she was anesthetized.

It is safest if a technician or another doctor monitors anesthesia while the veterinarian performs surgery: It's difficult to effectively focus on both patient monitoring and the surgical procedure at the same time.

Questions to ask:

- What kind of monitoring equipment is used for patients under anesthesia?
- Is a pulse oximeter attached to each patient to monitor oxygen levels?
- Is the equipment used during every anesthetic procedure, or only for certain patients?
- Who is monitoring the patient during anesthesia? Is there a veterinary technician assisting with anesthesia, or is the veterinarian alone with the patient while performing surgery?

---

6. Does the practice have licensed or experienced veterinary technicians?

The laws regarding veterinary technicians vary from state to state. Some states require veterinary technicians to be licensed, similar to a registered nurse for humans; others do not. Licensed technicians receive rigorous training in many areas, including how to properly measure and administer drugs, draw blood, place intravenous catheters, take radiographs, use anesthetic equipment, and monitor animals under anesthesia.

If your state requires licensing, check to see if the practice uses only licensed technicians. Even in states where this is not required by law, some practices will have licensed technicians. The more licensed technicians they have, the better for your pet. If the practice has unlicensed technicians, it is important to find out their level of experience, since they must learn their skills on the job rather than through formal training.

TIP The first step is to find out whether your state requires all veterinary technicians to be licensed. You can do this by calling the American Association of Veterinary State Boards at (877) 698-8482, or by going to their website, www.aavsb.org.

Questions to ask:

- If the state requires licensing of technicians: Do you use only licensed technicians?

- If the state does not require technicians to be licensed: Do you have any licensed technicians on staff?

- What is the level of training and experience level of any unlicensed technicians?

7. Is the practice AAHA-accredited?

As I discussed earlier, the American Animal Hospital Association (AAHA) provides voluntary accreditation to veterinary hospitals that meet stringent standards. AAHA accreditation provides you with assurance that the practice has met benchmarks in a variety of areas, including up-to-date facilities, equipment, patient care, and staffing. If there is an AAHA-accredited hospital in your area, this accreditation is a reassuring sign that the practice strives for a high standard of care.

Question to ask:

- Is the practice AAHA-accredited? (You can also check the AAHA website, www.healthypets.com.)

8. How many veterinarians are at the practice?

Although many wonderful veterinarians are solo practitioners, multidoctor practices may offer some advantages.

When there are several veterinarians in an office, your pet gets the benefit of the doctors' combined experience and knowledge. If a particular radiograph or test result is confusing, a veterinarian can confer with one or more of the other doctors, who may have encountered something similar or who are particularly skilled at interpretation. Additionally, different veterinarians have different areas of expertise. One may be adept at treating skin problems, another at surgery. Because it is difficult for any one practitioner to read every recent article or study and attend lectures on all the latest advances, you may feel more secure in going to a group where the doctors have complementary skill sets and knowledge.

In a group practice, there are also different levels of experience among the doctors, which can be an asset. More seasoned veterinarians are able to advise younger doctors; recent graduates, who tend to be very up-to-date on all the latest theories and technology, can help keep veterans on their toes. (Unfortunately, it is easy to quickly become obsolete in the practice of medicine, human or veterinary.) Unlike the situation in human medicine, veterinarians are not required to perform an internship after receiving their degrees, but can go straight into practice. Many do choose to undergo this valuable postgraduate training, however, and it is an advantage if any of the veterinarians at the practice have completed an internship program.

Some group practices have one or more board-certified specialists on staff, which is a bonus. Additionally, multidoctor practices are often able to afford more advanced equipment and a larger staff, such as overnight employees. They may have more extensive office hours as well.

Questions to ask:

- How many veterinarians are in your practice?
- Have any of the veterinarians completed an internship program?
- Are any of the veterinarians board-certified specialists? If so, in what areas?
- What are the office hours of the practice?

What if a practice does not pass every question?

The ideal practice would answer every question with flying colors, yet realistically you may not find one in your area that does so. Look for the practice that satisfies the highest number of these criteria, and also use your common sense and instincts to decide which practice seems to best meet the spirit of the standards we have discussed.

CHECKLIST: AT YOUR APPOINTMENT

If you are satisfied with the responses to the preliminary round of questions, you can use the following criteria to evaluate the practice during an appointment with or without your pet.

1. Is the practice clean and well organized?

In the practice of medicine, cleanliness is more than just cosmetic. It helps prevent the spread of infection and creates a more comfortable, less stressful environment for the patients. Attention to detail is key to effective patient care. Disorganization is more than just unsightly; it can be dangerous! Mix-ups with medication or test results can be life threatening to patients.

Take a look around the waiting area while you wait for your appointment to begin. Then look around the exam room. Additionally, ask to see where the hospitalized animals are kept (unless the staff are especially busy, they should be willing to take you there for a quick look). Pay particular attention to the following key factors:

- Does everything appear clean and tidy? Does it smell okay (within reason for an animal hospital)?

- Do the records and other paperwork at the front desk seem organized?

- Are the employees' uniforms clean and neat?

- In the exam room, are the table and equipment immaculate?

If they allow you to visit the hospitalized-patient area, ask yourself these questions:

- Is the area sanitary and well lit? Are the cages clean and dry, with some type of bedding or paper inside?

- Are the counters, tables, and floors clean and free of blood, urine, feces, uncapped needles, or used syringes?

2. Does the practice keep complete and detailed medical records?

Although there are specific laws that regulate proper medical record keeping, it's impossible for every veterinary practice to be monitored (except by pet owners themselves). But that doesn't mean that a practice can or should ignore the rules. Sloppy and/or incomplete medical records can indicate sloppy and/or incomplete medical care.

If medical records are not complete and detailed, there is no reason to assume that the patient's care was any better. Each time a pet is seen and examined, a full report of the findings should be entered in the medical record. The pet's symptoms should be noted, as well as other pertinent information from the owner. *All* physical exam findings should be listed, not just the abnormal ones. Different possible diagnoses, and the veterinarian's plan for obtaining a definitive diagnosis, should be outlined.

In contrast, merely jotting down a few lines of illegible chicken scratch is insufficient. It may save the doctor time, but it's not acceptable medical practice. Another veterinarian reading a patient's record should be able to easily understand everything that has happened in the animal's medical history, how the animal was treated, and why.

At the conclusion of your first appointment, you can ask for a copy of the record (or if you have been using the practice, you can request previous records). Owners are entitled to copies of their pet's complete medical records. You should receive every page, not selected ones. If you ask for the records, this request should be honored promptly and pleasantly (but don't expect the receptionist with ten clients in the waiting room to drop everything and start photocopying!). The copy should include your pet's entire medical file, including the doctor's handwritten or typed notes, physical exam findings, test results, surgery reports, and daily treatment sheets if your animal has been hospitalized. If any of these items appears to be missing, you can ask to review the original record, though you cannot take it off the premises. Don't worry if you can't understand all the medical terminology; you can still evaluate the records for completeness and organization.

Here are specific items to look for:

- Each time your pet was seen, a thorough medical history and complete physical exam should be recorded (see chapter 2).

- If your pet had surgery, the record should include a complete description of the procedure. For example, the veterinarian should record how the surgery was performed step-by-step, what kind of suture material was chosen, and which suturing technique was used.

- If your pet received medication, the record should clearly note the name of the medication, how much was dispensed, and for how long it was to be given.

- If your pet was hospitalized, the record should include daily treatment sheets with all fluids and medications given each day. If you are not sure what your animal received and want to make certain everything was properly recorded, you can compare the record with your bill, where it should all be itemized.

- For hospitalized patients, a daily physical examination, notes on the patient's progress, and the doctor's plan should be recorded *each day*.

- All test results should be included.

Many practices now use computerized medical records, which are not essential to practice excellent medicine but can be indicative of an up-to-date, organized practice. When choosing a practice, you can generally consider computerized medical records to be a positive sign.

3. Are prescription drugs dispensed properly and with appropriate monitoring?

It is crucial for your pet's health and safety that medications are properly stored, dispensed, and labeled. Sloppy or outdated drug-dispensing practices may reflect a sloppy or outdated practice of medicine.

Veterinarians should only dispense prescription drugs to patients they have examined relatively recently, even though pet owners would sometimes rather avoid the inconvenience or expense of an office visit. There are three primary reasons why you want your veterinarian to examine your pet before prescribing medication.

First, to the untrained eye, certain medical conditions can look very similar: a bacterial skin infection versus a fungal skin infection, or runny eyes due to allergies versus runny eyes due to a virus. In some situations, the wrong medication isn't just ineffective but can also be dangerous. For example, if an animal who has a viral infection in the eyes is given a steroid-containing eye ointment intended for allergies, the pet could suffer severe corneal damage or even blindness.

Second, animals who are not examined and monitored are more likely to experience side effects from medications. Thus, a reluctance to dispense medication without a recent office visit is a sign of a responsible veterinarian.

Third, there are laws against dispensing medication or prescriptions without a current veterinarian–client–patient relationship. So not only are periodic examinations of pets on medication essential for the patient's health, they are a legal requirement for veterinarians.

If you are evaluating a new practice, ask to see examples of how drugs are dispensed. Medications should always be dispensed in appropriate

---

Medication Side Effects

Patients who are taking certain medications long-term must be monitored carefully for side effects, often by periodic blood tests. Common examples of medications used for veterinary patients that require follow-up blood work are phenobarbital, enalapril (Vasotec, Enacard), carprofen (Rimadyl), and methimazole (Tapazole).

Phenobarbital is an anti-convulsant used to treat animals with seizures and can cause liver damage. Carprofen is an arthritis medication that can also affect the liver; enalapril is a heart medication that can affect kidney function. To protect the organs, patients on these medications require periodic blood tests to check for any changes.

Methimazole, an effective medication used to treat cats with overactive thyroid glands, can cause side effects in about one-third of the feline patients who take it. These include physical symptoms such as vomiting and itchiness, but also life-threatening conditions like anemia, decreased white blood cells, decreased platelet cells, liver toxicity, and decreased kidney function. To monitor for these changes, which can usually be reversed if caught early, it is imperative that cats taking methimazole have their blood tested about every three months.

If your veterinarian insists on monitoring patients who are taking these or other medications, this is a good sign! Rather than trying to make a fast buck, he is practicing responsible medicine. The practice that dispenses these medications continuously without requiring periodic blood work is not doing you a favor. Pet owners must also do their part by complying with monitoring recommendations. It is all too easy to let time slip by and put off making an appointment, putting your pet at unnecessary risk.

child-resistant containers (*not* paper envelopes!). In addition, the label should be complete, including:

- The name, address, and telephone number of the veterinarian.
- The pet owner's last name and the name of the pet.
- The date.
- The name, strength, and quantity of the medication.
- The dose and the duration of the course of medication.
- The expiration date of the medication.
- Any cautionary statements.

By contrast, you should be concerned if medications are dispensed with minimal labeling, in an inappropriate container, such as a little white envelope with "once a day" scrawled on it.

This may all sound like window dressing, but it is important for you and your pet, and not only because there are laws governing this area of veterinary medicine. Rather, if a practice has fallen behind in the way it dispenses drugs or monitors patients who are taking drugs, it may well have fallen behind in other important ways.

4. Does the practice use modern, aseptic surgical techniques?

When performing surgery, veterinarians should wear *all* of the following:

- Scrubs.
- Surgical mask.
- Surgical cap.
- *Sterile* gown.
- *Sterile* gloves.

If this protocol is not followed, your pet is put at higher risk of infection. In addition, failure to adhere to this standard may indicate a generally outdated or careless practice of medicine. During your appointment, ask the veterinarian what she wears when performing surgery. She should tell you she wears all five of the items listed above. Some veterinarians also wear shoe covers.

5. Are patients properly evaluated before anesthesia and surgery?

I recommend at a minimum the following criteria:

- All pets should have a physical exam within one month before undergoing anesthesia and surgery.

- Pets who are more than five years old should have blood work to evaluate organ function and assess anesthetic risk prior to the procedure.

We often find issues on a physical exam that are important to know about before anesthetizing a pet. For example, if a pet has a heart murmur, the anesthesia protocol must be modified, monitoring should be more intense, and a cardiologist may need to be consulted. An animal whose liver does not function normally can be endangered if certain types of drugs are used for sedation or anesthesia. An animal with kidney disease may suffer additional kidney damage during anesthesia if precautions are not taken.

Ask the veterinarian how the practice evaluates animals before anesthesia, in particular animals more than five years old.

6. Do patients receive proper pain management? Does the practice consider pain control an important issue?

Sadly, there was a time when pain medications were not widely used in veterinary medicine. Animals who had surgery or painful conditions often did not receive any medication to alleviate their suffering.

Today pain management is of major concern in veterinary medicine. Many new medications have been developed specifically for animals, and many medications once used solely to control pain in humans have been adopted for animals. Make sure that the practice where your pets are treated considers pain control an important issue, and do not automatically assume this is the case.

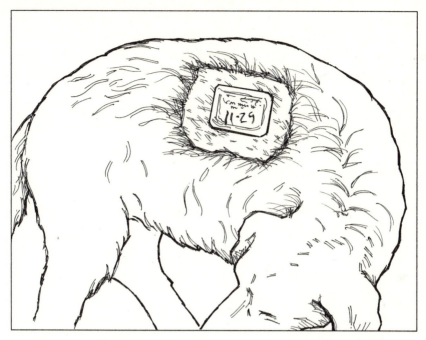

A dog with a pain-medication skin patch in place. The hair has been clipped to allow the patch to adhere.

A common example of when pain control is essential is when animals are spayed or neutered. In the immediate postoperative period, while still at the hospital, these animals should receive pain medication; once home, they should continue to take medication for several days. For animals having major surgery, this protocol is even more important. Following orthopedic surgery, for example, animals will need fairly aggressive pain control for days or even weeks.

Pain medications come in several forms. Generally, in the immediate postoperative period, while still hospitalized, animals will receive injections of narcotics or nonsteroidal anti-inflammatory drugs (NSAIDs) to control pain. When the animal goes home, the pain medication may be in the form of a pill, liquid, or sometimes a patch that is placed on the skin and releases medication for several days.

Ask the veterinarian about the practice's philosophy regarding pain control in animals. Generally, you will be able to ascertain during a brief discussion whether she considers this an important issue.

Inquire specifically whether animals undergoing elective surgery such as a spay (ovariohysterectomy) receive pain medication afterward. If the practice prioritizes pain control, the answer will be yes.

Pain Medications

Luckily, we now have many options for controlling pain in animals. One of the most convenient developments is the use of patches placed on the skin that release controlled amounts of medication for several days. These patches may contain a narcotic pain reliever or a local anesthetic.

As in human medicine, many new nonsteroidal anti-inflammatory medications are now available for animals. NSAIDs that are in the category called *COX-2 selective* are less likely to cause some of the side effects, such as stomach ulcers, that older NSAIDs were notorious for. However, even the newest NSAIDs can have side effects, including gastrointestinal ulceration. So pets who take them should be monitored carefully for signs of a problem, such as loss of appetite.

Check the types of pain medications used by the practice. If they have modern pain medications such as skin patches or the new COX-2 selective NSAIDs, this is a sign that the practice is focused on pain control and using current methods.

Hopefully all of the criteria we discussed in this chapter have helped you to better understand some of the elements that are important to consider when evaluating a veterinary practice. Of course, there are always those intangibles—a feeling of trust, a gentle manner, a willingness to go the extra mile—that are harder to quantify. If you find a practice that satisfies the objective measures discussed here as well as these intangible factors, you will be on your way to ensuring that you and your pet obtain the trusted care you both deserve.

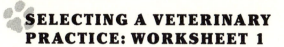

SELECTING A VETERINARY PRACTICE: WORKSHEET 1

Record the answers to your telephone questions here. Ideally, the answer to all the following questions should be yes. Realistically, you may have to accept the practice in your area with the highest score.

1. Are sick patients monitored at night or referred to a practice with overnight care?   Yes   No

2. Does the practice have equipment to measure blood pressure?   Yes   No

3. Does the practice have a PCV centrifuge or other equipment to measure red blood cell levels?   Yes   No

4. Does the practice have a pulse oximeter?   Yes   No

5. Does the practice use an automatic processor to develop X-rays (or have digital radiography)?   Yes   No

6. Does the practice refer patients to specialists?   Yes   No

7. Does the practice use isoflurane or sevoflurane gas anesthesia?   Yes   No

8. Do patients have an IV catheter placed before anesthesia?   Yes   No

9. Are patients intubated during anesthesia?   Yes   No

10. Are patients monitored with a pulse oximeter during anesthesia?   Yes   No

11. Does the practice have licensed or experienced veterinary technicians?   Yes   No

12. Is the practice AAHA-accredited?   Yes   No

13. Find out how many veterinarians are at the practice. Are you satisfied with the number?   Yes   No

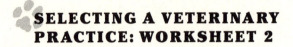

SELECTING A VETERINARY PRACTICE: WORKSHEET 2

Record information you learn about the practice during an appointment here.

1. Is the practice clean and well organized?	Yes	No
2. Does the practice keep complete and detailed medical records?	Yes	No
3. Are prescription drugs dispensed in childproof containers with complete labels?	Yes	No
4. Does the veterinarian wear scrubs, mask, cap, sterile gown, and sterile gloves when performing surgery?	Yes	No
5. Do patients more than five years old have blood tests before anesthesia and surgery?	Yes	No
6. Do patients receive proper pain management? Does the practice consider pain control to be an important issue?	Yes	No

CHAPTER 2

Head to Tail:

Making the Most of Your Pet's Appointments

I often think of a cat named Max I met years ago. When I saw him for the first time, he had barely been eating for months and had lost a lot of weight. Max really did look awful, and his family told me they were sure he had a fatal illness; they had brought him in for euthanasia. I began the appointment, as always, by taking a medical history, and learned that Max's only symptom was that he wouldn't eat. I asked the family if they would like me to do a physical exam and try to determine what was wrong with Max. They agreed, but it was obvious they felt there was no hope.

On Max's physical exam, I didn't find anything amiss except that he was terribly thin, a bit dehydrated, and had horrendous dental disease. His teeth were all loose and infected. His mouth was so sore that he was drooling constantly. I explained this to his family, and gently suggested we perform blood work and then do dentistry on Max if his organs were okay. They agreed, though they still seemed doubtful that Max had a chance. The blood work showed that Max's organs were fine, and the next day we put the cat under anesthesia and removed a number of loose, rotten, painful teeth. He ate a big meal that very afternoon; he was so relieved to have those mean old sore teeth gone! Max went home much happier, and

I received a thrilled call the next week from the family, telling me how wonderfully Max was doing—eating like a champ, and back to his old self.

This is a story not only about dental disease, but also about the importance of a detailed history and complete physical examination. In Max's case, when I questioned the family, there was no history of any symptoms other than his reluctance to eat. Certainly a poor appetite can be a sign of serious underlying disease, but a thorough physical exam revealed the probable cause, which was easily remedied. Had I rushed through the appointment, instead of listening carefully to what this family was telling me and performing a full physical exam, Max would have used up his ninth life unnecessarily. Of course, it is also a story about the importance of regular checkups: If Max had come in for a physical each year, his dental problems would have been discovered much earlier, sparing him a lot of pain and his family a lot of worry.

Having experienced it so many times with my own four-legged family, I can understand why a trip to the veterinarian's office is not necessarily the activity you and your pet most look forward to. Some dogs love car rides, adore everyone they meet, and forgive the veterinarian and her staff a variety of insults—thermometers in the most private areas, bitter-tasting pills and powders, and even surgery that leads to some missing anatomy. Other dogs and many cats are not quite so cooperative, and seem to know your evil plot hours in advance—like the dog who has to be forcibly dragged out from behind the sofa, and then looks at you as though you're turning him over to enemy agents when you (finally) get him into the car, and the cat who somehow manages to hide under the bed before you even get the carrier out. And anyone who has ever tried it knows that putting a cat in a carrier can be like trying to shove a panicked porcupine into a sock with your bare hands.

Then there's the car ride. It seems like it's always either pouring rain or at least ninety degrees outside. Your pet usually manages to get carsick within the first mile. You find yourself trying to clean it up with a crumpled old tissue while driving sixty miles an hour and making soothing noises. Dogs incessantly pant and drool, covering every surface in the car with gallons of sticky canine-scented saliva. Cats make horrible, heart-wrenching, tortured moans the entire ride until your nerves are as taut as violin strings.

It can be tempting to avoid all this entirely and skip your pet's yearly checkup. Or, if your pet is displaying potentially worrisome symptoms, you may put off taking him to the veterinarian because you so dread the whole experience or you feel guilty about the stress it seems to put him through. You wait and hope that the symptoms will just magically disappear.

As a veterinarian, I know how important it is to grit your teeth and bring in your pet for yearly checkups, or sooner if an animal is showing signs of a problem. I have seen the heartbreaking outcome when symptoms are ignored for too long. But as a pet owner, I understand how stressful a trip to the veterinarian can be, and how hard it is to even find the time. That's why I am so appreciative when my clients bring their pets in, and I feel it is my job to repay their efforts by giving them and their pets my full attention.

WHAT TO EXPECT AT EACH APPOINTMENT

Now that you've gotten your pet to the veterinarian's office, you want to be darn sure it's well worth the trouble. It's essential for your pet's health that the visit includes a complete physical examination as well as a series of questions called a *medical history* that enables the veterinarian to accurately assess your pet's condition. This can be a challenge. Appointment lengths vary from practice to practice, with many veterinarians seeing patients every fifteen or twenty minutes. The veterinarian's day can be a juggling act of outpatients, procedures, phone calls, and paperwork. While this is the reality of medical practice, it should not result in an abbreviated evaluation of your pet.

The exception would be a pet who has recently had a full exam and is in for some type of follow-up. For example, if your pet's blood tests show an abnormality, your veterinarian may recommend repeated blood work after fasting or a course of medication. A pet who has a splint or bandage may need to have it changed; a pet who has had surgery may need to have stitches removed. These types of visits may not require a full exam and history, since both have recently occurred.

Whether you are seeing the veterinarian for a routine checkup or because your pet has symptoms of illness, you'll want to get the most out of your appointment. You can help your pet by making sure that both the medical history and the physical exam are thorough and complete. Even if you are bringing your pet in for a specific problem, you don't want the veterinarian to skip any part of these two essential steps. By focusing exclusively on one symptom or part of the body, something vital to your pet's health could be missed.

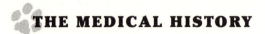

THE MEDICAL HISTORY

By understanding the topics that make up a proper medical history, you can help ensure that you and your veterinarian are communicating effectively about your pet's health. You can also use this knowledge to help you evaluate the quality of care at a veterinary practice. The medical history is a series of questions a doctor asks to make sure she has all the pertinent information about the patient. Even during a routine checkup, problems are often uncovered through the history. Each of the following topics should be covered during your pet's exam. The first two questions will only need to be discussed the first time your pet sees a new doctor, since the answers will not change. The other questions should be discussed during each appointment.

1. How long have you had this pet?

If you have had your pet since she was very young, the veterinarian can assume that you know everything that has happened in her life, including any previous health problems. If your pet was an adult when you brought her home, there may be unknown aspects to her health history or events that occurred before she lived with you. Without knowing when you got your pet, the veterinarian could miss helpful clues.

For example, some pets develop respiratory problems from being exposed to secondhand smoke. If I see a pet who has been coughing, I always ask the owners if they smoke. If they say no, I might assume that I'm on the wrong track—unless I discover, for example, that until recently the pet lived with an elderly aunt who was a chain-smoker. By always asking how long a client has had a pet, I make sure not to miss this type of valuable information.

When pets are obtained as adults, sometimes their exact age is unknown. Yet the pet's age may affect how the veterinarian interprets certain findings or which tests he runs, so be sure to let him know if your pet's age is in question. For example, cats over the age of seven can develop overactive thyroid glands. Say your cat was an adult stray when you adopted her

The Story of Sheba

I once treated a beautiful dog named Sheba whose owners were worried because she was losing weight and had unusual abnormalities on her blood tests. During the history, I learned Sheba was originally from Greece, where her owners had found her during their vacation. Because of this, I suspected she had a chronic infection called leishmaniasis that is more common in Greece than in the United States. When I tested her bone marrow, where the infection is often found, sure enough, the *Leishmania* organisms were there.

several years ago, and at that time you guessed she was two years old—when in fact she was five. If your cat now has unexplained weight loss, your veterinarian might not think to test her thyroid level if he doesn't realize that her age is just an estimate.

2. Where did you get your pet?

A pet's background can yield important clues to any problems that may crop up. For example, a puppy purchased at a pet store may be more likely to have infectious diseases (such as kennel cough) or intestinal parasites (such as coccidia or *Giardia*). A dog from the Midwest is more likely to have certain fungal infections than one from the East Coast, and a dog brought to the United States from another country can have health issues not normally seen here.

3. Has your pet ever traveled out of the area?

Similarly, pets who have traveled may be carrying infections not typically seen in your hometown or region. This includes travel to another continent, another state, or even out of the city for a weekend trip to the country. If your veterinarian isn't aware that your pet has traveled, he may not consider these infections. Even if the travel took place years ago, it may still be relevant.

For example, ehrlichiosis is an infectious disease transmitted by ticks in certain parts of the world, and dogs can carry this disease for years before it is diagnosed. Knowing your dog has traveled to one of the areas where the disease is prevalent will tip off your veterinarian to test for it.

4. Has your pet had any previous health issues?

This question will be especially important if you are visiting a new veterinary practice. Hopefully, you will have copies of your pet's previous records to give to your new veterinarian, but it is always helpful to briefly discuss prior medical conditions. Even something that seems insignificant to you may be relevant. Also, be sure to let the veterinarian know if your pet has ever had a bad reaction to a medicine or vaccine.

5. What do you feed your pet?

The exam is an opportunity for you and your veterinarian to discuss a healthy diet that is appropriate for your pet, and to remedy an unbalanced diet before it causes problems.

A common mistake, for instance, is to feed a dog only meat, which is very low in calcium. Dogs who eat only meat, instead of dog food or a balanced homemade diet, are at risk of bone weakness, among other problems. In fact, their bones can become so fragile that the animal suffers multiple fractures.

One worrying situation that I sometimes encounter during exams is an owner who tells me that her cat likes to eat the dog's food. Because dog food does not have enough taurine (see the sidebar) for a cat, the cat is at risk for developing heart disease as well as blindness. By taking a thorough history, I can discover this situation and warn the owner of the danger before it is too late.

Cat Food and Taurine

In the 1980s, a veterinary cardiologist named Dr. Paul Pion discovered that a deficiency of the amino acid taurine in cat food was causing thousands of cats to go into heart failure. Humans and dogs can manufacture this amino acid in their bodies, but cats cannot, even though they need more than other species.

Taurine is found naturally only in animal tissue. Because cats evolved as pure carnivores living on prey, they never had a need to make this amino acid, so they never developed the ability to produce it themselves. After Dr. Pion's discovery, taurine was added to cat food, and the devastating heart disease called feline dilated cardiomyopathy virtually disappeared.

The Story of Bellina

When I noticed that my own cat Bellina was eating more than usual without gaining any weight, I suspected that something was wrong. I ran tests and discovered she had a type of cancer called lymphoma in her intestines. The cancer was affecting her intestinal function so that she was unable to absorb nutrients, causing her to feel hungry all the time. By diagnosing it quickly, I was able to treat her with medication, giving her four more happy years.

New advances in animal nutrition are happening all the time. Every year, we know more about the healthiest ways to feed pets. The exam is an opportunity for the veterinarian to share this new information.

6. How is your pet's appetite?

A decreased appetite is a common symptom of a variety of health problems—an alarm signal that something may be seriously wrong. If your pet is eating less than he used to, the cause should be investigated.

On the other hand, an increased appetite can indicate certain hormonal or digestive problems, and also should not be ignored. Some diseases, such as Cushing's disease (an excess of steroid hormones), cause pets to eat more and gain weight. Others, like diabetes, an overactive thyroid, or digestive problems, may cause a pet to eat more yet lose weight. Either is cause for concern.

7. How much water does your pet drink? Is your pet drinking more than she used to?

If your pet is drinking more water than she used to, this can indicate a hormonal imbalance, a kidney problem, certain infections, or other issues.

For example, dogs and cats who are not spayed can develop a severe infection in their uterus called pyometra. One of the first symptoms is increased thirst due to bacterial toxins. This infection is life threatening if untreated, and, similar to an inflamed appendix in people, the infected uterus can rupture. It is essential to diagnose pyometra as early as possible.

If your pet is drinking more water than she used to, your veterinarian will want to run tests to find out why. Conditions that cause excessive thirst can be serious, but many are treatable if diagnosed promptly.

8. Is your pet urinating normally?

Abnormal urination may include larger amounts of urine (which often occurs when the pet is drinking more water), more frequent urination, urination in inappropriate places, straining to urinate, or an abnormal appearance to the urine (such as blood or discoloration).

> TIP An animal's urinary tract can become completely obstructed, which is a life-threatening emergency. The blockage may be due to urinary stones or other causes. This condition is most common in male cats, but can happen in any dog or cat. If your pet is having extreme difficulty urinating or attempting to urinate without success, he must see a veterinarian immediately.

If your pet's urinations change in any way, your vet will need to look for underlying medical causes. If a pet urinates in inappropriate places, the owner sometimes assumes that the pet is misbehaving when there is actually a medical reason, such as a bladder infection, bladder stone, or even diabetes.

If your pet is having any urinary problems, bring a urine sample with you to your appointment. Be sure to use a clean container, and try to catch the urine midstream, before it hits the ground. Your veterinarian may want to obtain a sterile urine sample by cystocentesis, which involves taking urine from the bladder with a needle. This procedure, which may sound scary but is actually routine, is the preferred method of obtaining urine, especially when diagnosing urinary tract infections.

> TIP Try not to let your pet urinate right before your appointment with the veterinarian. This way, if the veterinarian wants to obtain a sterile sample, the bladder will not be empty. To prevent a small dog from urinating, you may want to carry him in your arms. If you have a larger dog, try to keep him from stopping and sniffing. In case you're unable to prevent your dog from urinating on the way, bring a clean container with you so that you can collect a sample. If your pet is a cat, there isn't an easy way to prevent her from urinating in the carrier.

9. Is your pet coughing or sneezing?

Either one of these symptoms can signal a problem. Coughing can be caused by viral or bacterial infections, allergic bronchitis, parasites, tra-

The Story of Bobby

I often think of a cat called Bobby that I once treated. His owner had tearfully brought Bobby to the practice because her husband, upset that the cat had been urinating outside his litter box, was insisting that Bobby be given away. The problem had been going on for months, and the owner had assumed it was a behavioral issue. When we took radiographs, we found the cause of all the trouble: a large bladder stone! Once Bobby's stone was removed, he felt much better, and the problem was solved.

cheal (windpipe) abnormalities, heart disease, tumors, and more. Coughing in a cat can also be a sign of asthma, which if untreated can cause lung damage and trouble breathing. Owners often assume some coughing is normal in cats, but in fact healthy cats rarely cough. They may also think that the cat is simply trying to cough up a hairball when in fact he's having an asthma attack.

Sneezing can be mild and insignificant, or more severe and a sign of conditions such as viral or fungal infections, tumors, or even objects lodged in the nasal cavity. When due to more serious conditions, sneezing is usually accompanied by nasal discharge.

10. Is your pet vomiting?

Vomiting occurs for many reasons, and the causes range from minor issues to very serious diseases. If your pet is vomiting, you and your veterinarian should promptly investigate the cause.

Cats do tend to vomit more than dogs. For instance, cats will occasionally vomit hairballs or regurgitate when they eat too fast. This type of vomiting, if infrequent, can be normal. However, if your cat is vomiting more than he used to, it may be a sign of a serious problem, especially if the vomiting is combined with unexplained weight loss. Unfortunately, since they tend to vomit more than other animals, cats with conditions that cause vomiting sometimes do not receive treatment until the disease is quite advanced.

If your pet is vomiting, your veterinarian will ask you a few questions that will help determine if it is true vomiting or actually regurgitation; because the two have different causes, it is important to determine which one is happening. It is a common error to confuse regurgitation with vomiting, which can make it more difficult to reach a diagnosis. True vomiting is a more forceful act, and the abdomen will contract, or heave. Regurgitation is passive; there are no abdominal contractions, and the animal often brings up undigested food, sometimes in a tubular shape.

11. Has your pet had any diarrhea?

Diarrhea can be caused by many factors, including diet, parasites, infections, digestive problems, and more. Everybody gets diarrhea once in a while (especially when we eat something we shouldn't!), but more frequent or persistent diarrhea should be addressed.

If your pet has diarrhea, your veterinarian will ask you a series of questions to pinpoint whether it's caused by a problem with the small intestine, the large intestine (colon), or both. This helps determine the cause of the diarrhea, the seriousness of the condition, and what therapy should be used.

Questions that will help localize the problem to the large intestine include:

- Does the stool contain any mucus or blood?

- Does your pet have increased urgency to defecate? The pet may need to defecate more frequently or have accidents in the house.

- Does your pet strain or show discomfort when defecating?

Questions that will help localize the problem to the small intestine include:

- Is your pet losing weight? Since nutrients are absorbed in the small intestine, weight loss may occur if the diarrhea is due to disease of the small intestine. Weight loss also tends to indicate a more serious problem.

- Are there unusually large amounts of stool?

- Does the pet's stomach growl? This is called borborygmus.

- Is the stool an unusual color, such as paler than usual or black? Lighter or clay-colored stools can indicate a problem with digestion or intestinal absorption; black, tarry stools can indicate bleeding in the small intestine or stomach.

If your pet has had diarrhea, bring a recent stool sample with you. The sample should be in a clean container, and should be refrigerated (yes, ugh) until your appointment.

12. Has your pet lost or gained weight?

TIP Weight loss is often the first indication of a problem, yet it's often overlooked. You should keep an eye on your pet's weight and alert your veterinarian of any unexplained weight loss immediately. Each time your pet is seen, be sure to ask your veterinarian to compare the current weight with the previous one. Sometimes when an older pet is losing weight, the owner assumes the change is due to aging. Aging alone will not cause a pet to lose weight, however; an underlying illness should be suspected if this occurs.

Your veterinarian will weigh your pet at every appointment, and then compare the most recent with the previous weight. If this is your first time at a new practice, the veterinarian should ask you if your pet's weight is stable. Unless the pet has been on a weight-reduction program, weight loss is a red flag that something may be seriously wrong.

Weight gain is an even more common problem for our pets, and your doctor will want to investigate whether it is due to a health issue, such as a hormonal imbalance, or simply overfeeding. Besides being a symptom of certain illnesses, weight gain can also lead to problems like diabetes or worsening of arthritis. Obesity is a serious issue for American pets, and if necessary, your veterinarian can counsel you on a safe weight-loss program for your pet.

13. Do you give your pet any medications or supplements?

Depending on the season and the area you live in, your veterinarian may ask you if your pet receives preventives against heartworms, fleas, and ticks. Heartworm disease is an easily preventable infection that is fatal in dogs if untreated. Many people are not aware that cats can also be infected by heartworms, and that in many areas of the country they, too, should receive preventive medication.

Fleas not only are irritating to the pet but can also cause severe skin conditions and anemia. It may come as a surprise to hear that fleas can actually kill an animal due to blood loss (fleas live on blood from the animals they infest). Ticks carry multiple diseases, which are called tick-borne infections (such as Lyme disease, Rocky Mountain spotted fever, and ehrlichiosis), so it is essential to protect pets who go outdoors from tick bites.

If you are seeing a new veterinarian, she will ask if your pet is taking any other medications, such as nonsteroidal anti-inflammatory drugs (NSAIDs). Animals who take NSAIDs, often for arthritis, must be monitored carefully for side effects, and these medications should not be given with certain other drugs or to animals with some medical conditions. Be sure to tell your veterinarian about any medications your pet is taking.

TIP *Never* give your dog or cat any medication without first speaking to your veterinarian. Many over-the-counter or human medications can be extremely toxic to animals, particularly cats.

Your veterinarian will also want to know if you give your pet any vitamins, herbs, or supplements. Pet owners are not always aware of the side effects that these can have; people often assume that anything from the health food store must be harmless, which unfortunately is not true. For example, the common herb ginseng can cause high blood pressure, headache, vomiting, tremors, and sleeplessness. The herb ma huang causes a dangerously rapid heart rate, high blood pressure, tremors, and seizures, and has been fatal to animals. Certain vitamins and minerals such as iron, vitamin A, and vitamin D can be toxic at inappropriate doses.

The Story of Pretzel

Several years ago I took care of a little dog named Pretzel who almost died of liver damage due to vitamins. Pretzel had become very ill, and tests showed that his liver was failing. During the medical history, we discovered that the owner had recently adopted two children who needed vitamins due to previous malnutrition. The children did not like taking their vitamins, so they would sometimes give them to Pretzel. The owner did not realize that, at the wrong dose, vitamins could be very dangerous. The iron in the vitamins was toxic to Pretzel, and his liver began to fail. Luckily, once we pinpointed the problem and treated him, he made a full recovery.

What if my pet has other symptoms?

Of course the list above does not include every symptom an animal can have. It only includes the basic topics that should be covered during every appointment. You may have made the appointment because of an abnormality you noticed, such as limping, bad breath, decreased vision, or something else that concerned you. Be sure to tell your veterinarian about any changes you have noticed in your pet, even something as subtle as a decreased energy level.

🐾 GETTING THE MOST OUT OF YOUR APPOINTMENT

If you're thinking, *Wow! That's a lot to talk about in a fifteen- or twenty-minute appointment*—you're right. That's why it's important to help your veterinarian (and your pet) by being efficient. Be sure to arrive about fifteen minutes early to check in. You don't want to waste precious appointment time that should be focused on your pet because you are late or cut it so close that a portion of your allotted time is spent doing paperwork.

To maximize your time with the veterinarian during the appointment, try to stick to the point and avoid going off on tangents or telling stories about your pet that are interesting but don't really contain essential information. When the veterinarian asks you a question, try to answer it concisely.

Try also to answer the questions as precisely as possible, especially when they concern how long your pet has been showing signs of illness. If your veterinarian asks you how long Felix has been sneezing or Bowser has been drinking more water, be specific: "About two weeks" is much clearer than "Awhile," which could mean days, weeks, or months.

Your answers should be truthful and complete, even if you are worried the veterinarian may disapprove of something. When I ask owners what their pets eat, the first answer may be "Dog food," but eventually it comes out that although Dixie does eat a little dog food, she also eats hot dogs, fried chicken, pork chops, and sometimes the garbage. Don't make the veterinarian waste time puzzling over why Dixie has diarrhea!

I often tell clients that my exam room is like a confessional, where they can feel comfortable telling the absolute truth. You will find that while veterinarians will offer constructive advice, we are rarely judgmental. Believe me, we've heard it all.

THE PHYSICAL EXAM

The next section will be a little like the first year of veterinary school, when we learned about anatomy. I will tell you everything you need to know about the components of a complete physical exam on a dog or cat. I'll go through the exam in the order that most veterinarians tend to perform it, but what's important is that nothing is left out. This way you can ensure that your pet receives a full physical while evaluating the thoroughness of the veterinarian's exam.

I'll also explain orthopedic and neurological examinations, which are generally performed only if the pet is having symptoms of a problem.

1. Eyes

The veterinarian will look at your pet's eyes, often with a penlight to be sure the pupils are working properly.

Ideally, your veterinarian should perform a fundic exam by using a lens to look at the retina, the lining at the back of the eye. This only takes a few seconds to perform, and is helpful in uncovering clues to the animal's overall health. If an animal has high blood pressure, for example, there may be changes in the retina that serve as clues. If the high blood pressure is not corrected, permanent blindness may occur.

2. Ears

The veterinarian will look into your pet's ears to check for infection or discharge. He may use an otoscope (a lighted instrument) to look farther into the ear canal if he suspects a problem.

3. Nose

The veterinarian will glance at the nose to check for discharge. If your animal has a history of sneezing, nasal discharge, or nosebleeds, the nasal exam will be more extensive.

4. Mouth

The veterinarian will open your pet's mouth to look for any abnormalities. She will check under the tongue and examine the teeth and gums to check for tartar, gingivitis, or infection.

Animals who tend to growl or bite may be muzzled, which makes it difficult for the doctor to properly examine the mouth. If they have had oral symptoms, such as drooling, difficulty chewing, or halitosis (bad breath), these pets may need to be sedated to allow the doctor a better look.

5. Lymph nodes

While some lymph nodes are hidden inside the body, others can be felt externally in several locations. The veterinarian will examine the lymph nodes under the chin (submandibular), in front of the shoulders (prescapular), in the armpits (axillary), in the groin (inguinal), and on the back of the thighs (popliteal). She wants to make sure none of the lymph nodes are enlarged.

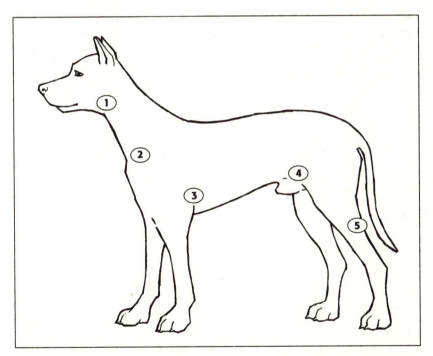

The external lymph nodes. In each location, there is a pair of lymph nodes, one on each side of the animal: 1. submandibular; 2. prescapular; 3. axillary; 4. inguinal; and 5. popliteal.

TIP Sometimes owners will notice at home that their pet has enlarged lymph nodes, especially those under the jaw, which may be felt when the owner is petting the animal. If you notice lumps under the chin or anywhere else on your pet, you should schedule an appointment with your veterinarian right away.

6. Skin

The veterinarian will run his hands over your pet's body to feel for any bumps, fleas, ticks, or rashes. If you have felt any skin bumps at home, it is good to point them out, since it is difficult for the doctor to examine every inch of your pet, and tiny bumps can be difficult to detect under the fur.

TIP Even very small skin bumps can be concerning and should be examined by your veterinarian. It's a good idea to dot the fur over the bump with a nontoxic marker before heading out the door. Just like when your car stops making that annoying clanging noise as soon as you reach the mechanic, the tiny bump will be impossible to find once you're at the doctor's office.

7. Heart and lungs

The veterinarian will listen to your pet's heart and lungs with a stethoscope to check for murmurs (abnormal noises during the heartbeat) or arrhythmias (abnormal heart rhythms), and to make sure the animal's lungs sound clear.

8. Abdomen

The veterinarian will feel your pet's abdomen to make sure none of the organs feel enlarged or abnormal, there are no masses inside the abdomen, and there is no evidence of fluid in the abdominal cavity.

I think that owners must sometimes wonder why I spend so much time apparently massaging their pet's belly. Especially in small animals, a careful veterinarian can often feel the kidneys, intestines, bladder, and enlargement of the liver or spleen.

9. Rectal examination

A rectal examination should be performed on every adult dog, and any dog with abnormal defecation. In male dogs, it is important to feel the prostate during each checkup.

Most cats will not allow a rectal examination without sedation. So unless there are symptoms that suggest a problem in the rectal area (such as blood on the stool or straining to defecate), this part of the physical exam is often skipped in cats.

10. Orthopedic examination

If your pet has been limping or stiff, the veterinarian will perform an orthopedic examination. This involves watching the pet walk, and then feeling each limb joint by joint for pain or swelling.

11. Neurological examination

If your pet has shown any symptoms that can indicate a possible neurological problem, such as poor balance, a tendency to bump into things, seizures, or paralysis, your veterinarian will perform a full neurological examination.

This includes checking the nerves of the head (cranial nerves), and also checking the function and reflexes of the limbs. To evaluate the cranial nerves, the veterinarian will check the animal's vision, the ability to blink, the response of the pupils to light, facial sensation, and eye movements. To evaluate the nerves supplying the spine and limbs, the veterinarian will check the animal's gait, strength, and reflexes, and manipulate the paws to see if the animal seems aware of the paw's position.

How can I help during the physical exam?

As you did with the history, you can help your veterinarian perform a more complete and efficient physical exam. If you have noticed apparent problems with your pet, tell your veterinarian. Try to be concise and accurate. For example, if your pet has been limping, pay attention to which leg is affected. Write it down so you won't have trouble remembering during your appointment.

TIP When we ask owners if the animal's right or left side has been affected, they sometimes find this confusing. If you are not sure, stand behind your pet. When you are looking at your pet from behind, facing the same direction as your pet, the animal's left and right are the same as yours.

If you have noticed an abnormality, such as a lump, your veterinarian will want to know how long it has been there and if it is changing. For example, your dog may have had the same little skin bump that has not grown at all for several years. Or the bump may be new and growing rapidly. Try to think about these kinds of things *before* your appointment so your time with the doctor can be used most effectively.

During the exam, you can help by calming your pet and, if possible, keeping her still. If your pet tends to growl or snap, or is just very wiggly, the veterinarian may have a technician restrain her; in this case, you can probably help most by staying out of the way unless they ask for your help.

Sometimes owners want to comfort their pets during the exam by hugging them or picking them up. Remember that if you are hugging your pet, the doctor may have trouble performing an exam. Try not to encourage or allow your pet to climb into your arms. Instead, stay by your pet's head, but leave her body free for the doctor to approach. Also, when the doctor is listening with the stethoscope, you'll want to be very quiet so he can hear your pet's heart and lungs clearly.

What can I do to prepare for my pet's appointment?

Before your appointment, get organized. You can use the medical history worksheet at the end of this chapter to prepare. Try to write down the answer to every question as well as any other symptoms you have seen. Be as specific as possible. For example, if your pet has been vomiting, how often does it occur? Once a week? Once a month? If your pet has been drinking more, how long has this been going on, and how severe is it? Has she been drinking just a little more water, or three times as much?

Make a list of any questions you would like to ask your veterinarian. We all know how easy it is to forget something you wanted to talk about. If you have been to another veterinarian with this pet, bring the medical records with you. Your old receipts are not the same as the medical records; you will need to ask the previous veterinarian to mail or fax a copy of the record to you. It is helpful if you can bring a copy for the new veterinarian to keep so time is not wasted during your appointment making photocopies. If you can't bring an extra copy, arrive early and ask the receptionist to make a copy.

Your goal is to have all of your appointment time devoted to discussing and examining your pet. You don't want to waste any of this time checking in, copying records, trying to remember which brand of food you buy, or calling home to ask someone to read the names of medications off the bottles. You are paying a doctor to focus on your pet for the length of your appointment. By being organized and efficient, you will get the most for your money and your pet's well-being. You may save yourself another trip, too. There are times when a client is so late or the appointment takes so long that if we need to do something such as take radiographs, we have to schedule another appointment.

TIP If you are taking your pet for an exam and you have noticed any unusual symptoms, the doctor may want to perform blood work or other tests on your pet. If this is the case, do not feed your pet (water is fine) for eight hours before your appointment. (Some animals should not be fasted, so check with your doctor if your pet is diabetic or very young, small, or weak.) Fasting will make the test results more accurate and allow your pet to be sedated, if necessary, for a test or procedure. This may also save you and your pet a return visit, as some blood tests can be performed only after fasting.

What should I do if I feel uncomfortable with something during the appointment?

If anything happens during the exam that makes you uncomfortable, calmly say so. If you are concerned for your pet's safety, ask the veterinarian to stop the proceedings and discuss your concerns. If you still have reservations after the conversation, tell her that you would like to leave with your pet. If your concerns are serious—you feel your pet was handled too roughly, for instance—you should find another practice where you are more comfortable.

Keep in mind that the veterinarian and her staff will have to be firm with an animal who may harm himself or others. It is common and acceptable to restrain a cat who is squirmy or upset while on the exam table by holding the skin at the scruff of his neck. A dog who growls or snaps will need to be muzzled. But if you feel that the handling of your pet is dangerous or unnecessarily rough or frightening, speak up and, if necessary, leave.

During the exam, your veterinarian should not give your pet any medication or vaccinations without first discussing it with you. If your veterinarian is preparing to give your pet an injection, ask him to stop and explain what it is, and why it's being given. If you do not feel comfortable with the explanation, do not hesitate to ask questions or even refuse the injection. At all points during your pet's appointment, it should be clear what is occurring, and you should be comfortable with the proceedings. At the conclusion of the visit, you should feel that your pet has been thoroughly examined and that all of your concerns have been addressed.

YOUR PET'S MEDICAL HISTORY: WORKSHEET

Make a copy of this worksheet to fill out and bring with you to your appointment. All questions should be covered. Write in the answers at home. At the appointment, check off the box when each topic is discussed.

Questions to Be Covered by Vet	Notes to Discuss with Vet	Covered During Visit?
How long have you had your pet?		☐
Where did you get your pet?		☐
Has your pet ever traveled out of the area? Where?		☐
Has your pet had any previous health issues?		☐
What do you feed your pet (include treats and snacks)?		☐
How is your pet's appetite?		☐

Questions to Be Covered by Vet	Notes to Discuss with Vet	Covered During Visit?
Is your pet drinking normally? Is your pet drinking more or less than usual?		☐
Are your pet's urinations normal? If not, how are they abnormal?		☐
Is your pet coughing or sneezing? Does he have nasal discharge?		☐
Is your pet vomiting? If so, is it true vomiting or regurgitation?		☐
Has your pet had any diarrhea? If yes, is there blood or mucus on it?		☐
Has your pet lost or gained weight since the last appointment?		☐
Is your pet on any medications or supplements?		☐

Questions to Be Covered by Vet	Notes to Discuss with Vet	Covered During Visit?
Are there any other problems or questions you want to discuss?		☐

PHYSICAL EXAM: WORKSHEET

Bring a copy of this with you to your appointment. The first nine areas should be examined at every checkup, the last two will be necessary only in pets displaying specific symptoms. Check off the box once the area has been examined, and note any abnormalities the veterinarian finds.

Examination Area	Covered by Vet?	Notes
1. Eyes, including fundic exam	☐	
2. Ears	☐	
3. Nose	☐	
4. Mouth	☐	
5. Lymph nodes	☐	
6. Skin and fur	☐	
7. Heart and lungs	☐	
8. Abdomen	☐	
9. Rectal exam (adult dog)	☐	

Examination Area	Covered by Vet?	Notes
10. Orthopedic exam (pet who is stiff or limping)	☐	
11. Neurological exam (pet displaying possible neurological symptoms)	☐	

Additional Notes from Exam

_____

_____

_____

_____

_____

_____

CHAPTER 3

Give It Your Best Shot:

Creating a Personalized Vaccination Protocol

Vaccination is a hot topic right now in both human and veterinary medicine. The risks and benefits of various vaccines for people and animals are under discussion by health care professionals, parents, and pet owners. In this chapter, we'll take a look at the present state of veterinary understanding in this area—including an overview of what we do and don't know—discuss some of the issues you may be concerned about, and formulate guidelines to help you make informed decisions about your pet's vaccination program.

There is much heated debate regarding vaccines, and it can be pretty tough to wade through all the rhetoric and hype to figure out what's actually the best plan for your pet. You may have seen information on the Internet that seems to contradict what your veterinarian recommends. I know that many of you aren't sure who to believe anymore; you hear all kinds of dire warnings about the perils of overvaccination, but you don't want to leave your companion unprotected, either. If you're like most people, you aren't even really sure which vaccines are available for dogs and cats, or which diseases they are supposed to be guarding against.

In the old days, people obediently brought their pets in for yearly shots. Now pet owners are questioning the number of vaccines that animals are given and the frequency of recommended booster injections. These are valid concerns that are also being discussed within the veterinary profession. We'll review our current knowledge regarding the ideal timing of booster shots, and we'll also talk about how vaccine protocols can (and should) be tailored for individual pets with differing environments and lifestyles.

It's important to recognize that the development of vaccines was an incredible medical milestone: The value of vaccinations for people and animals cannot be overemphasized. In a society where we don't even think about kids getting polio, we may be tempted to forget that not long ago, many thousands of children and adults were paralyzed due to infection with this virus. After the vaccine was introduced in 1955, the incidence of polio has decreased 99 percent worldwide, with the Americas free of polio since 1994. The disease may soon be eradicated, as smallpox was in 1977. Before that time, smallpox killed many millions of people, including three hundred to five hundred million in the twentieth century alone. Now the disease no longer exists, thanks to vaccination.

There have also been remarkable achievements through animal vaccination programs. In September 2007, for example, the Centers for Disease Control (CDC) announced that the United States was free of canine rabies. Although an unvaccinated dog is still at risk of infection from a wild animal, the strain generally transmitted from dog to dog (and then from dog to human) has been eliminated in this country. This situation is fragile, however, and can quickly change if we relax our vigilance. In parts of the world where widespread vaccination of dogs against rabies is not performed, the disease is common, with tragic consequences for both dogs and humans.

We must be very careful not to take vaccination for granted or to allow ourselves to be convinced not to vaccinate our pets. Those who choose not to vaccinate are putting their animals' lives at great risk, as well as the lives of other animals in the community. I think that those who speak out against vaccines must never have seen a puppy die from parvovirus, or a kitten from distemper. I have, all too often. The issue is not *whether* to vaccinate our pets, but with which vaccines and how often. As we go on, we'll answer these questions more specifically.

Is there such a thing as overvaccination?

Absolutely. There are certain vaccines that every dog or cat should receive, and others that only certain pets need depending on environment and lifestyle. If a pet were to be vaccinated against a disease that was not a danger to that particular animal, or were to be given vaccines more frequently than necessary, that could be considered overvaccination. On the other hand, there is even more risk associated with undervaccination, so it would be a mistake to avoid vaccinating your pet properly due to a general fear of vaccines.

How do vaccines work?

The word *vaccine* comes from the Latin *vacca,* meaning "cow." In 1796, Edward Jenner used an inoculation of cowpox to successfully immunize a young boy against smallpox infection, after noting that those who worked with cows seemed protected from smallpox, and more specifically that people who became infected with cowpox (a more mild viral infection with the Latin name *vaccinia*) did not contract the deadlier smallpox virus.

Vaccines are agents that protect the vaccinated individual by giving the immune system advance warning. Some vaccinations can prevent a disease entirely; others lessen the severity of illness when exposure occurs. There are many types of vaccines, generally containing all or part of a microorganism that has been rendered safe in some manner. For example, vaccines may contain killed microorganisms or microorganisms that are alive but disabled. Some contain inactivated toxins, to protect against illness caused by these toxins (as is the case with tetanus, or the new rattlesnake vaccine for dogs). Newer kinds of vaccines include recombinant types, where genes from the infectious agent are inserted into another (more harmless) virus.

Why are booster shots necessary?

There are excellent reasons to properly booster your pet's vaccinations. One of the most important for puppies and kittens is called maternally derived antibodies. When animals are born, they obtain temporary antibodies against infectious illnesses from their mother, mainly via the earliest milk, which is called colostrum. This occurs during the first day of life, after which the antibodies can no longer be absorbed by the intestinal tract. The amount of antibodies acquired against various diseases will vary depending on the mother's vaccination and disease history, and how much colostrum the newborn receives. These maternal antibodies offer some protection but also interfere with the action of vaccines by attacking the vaccinated agent before the young animal has time to mount a proper immune response. Until the maternally derived antibodies fade, vaccines are not fully effective.

The waning of maternal antibodies is unpredictable and can take up to four months to occur, so vaccine boosters should ideally be repeated until the puppy or kitten is around four months old. Since very young animals are especially vulnerable to infectious disease, and both the amount and duration of maternal antibodies are variable, we can't wait until this point to begin protecting them. For example, maternal antibodies may be lost by six weeks of age, or may last for sixteen weeks. Therefore, we initiate vaccines at around eight weeks of age (sometimes even earlier in high-risk situations) and then repeat them every three to four weeks until the four-month point when we know the maternally derived antibodies should be gone, so the vaccines can have long-lasting effects. This means that most puppies and kittens should be vaccinated three times: at around eight, twelve, and sixteen weeks of age.

For adult animals, booster vaccinations are used to restimulate fading immunity to a particular disease. The value and ideal timing of these boosters is currently under active investigation. Traditionally, vaccines were repeated each year, but this was fairly arbitrary and not based on scientific evidence of necessity. The veterinary profession is working very hard right now to figure out just how often each vaccine does need to be given to maintain good immunity. Although many veterinarians no longer believe that every vaccine must be repeated each year, the risk of decreasing the frequency too drastically is the danger of a sharp increase in fatalities from infectious illnesses. Although prior insistence on yearly vaccination aroused suspicion in the public and eroded trust in the veterinary profession, a resultant backlash away from vaccination could have devastating consequences.

It is important to maintain immunity not only in individual animals, but also in the community; the more immunity present in the population, the safer each animal is. To understand this concept, think about whether you would feel safer sending your child to a school where all the children were properly vaccinated and infectious illness was rare, or one in which few children were vaccinated and disease was common. Or consider the examples of smallpox and polio: By properly vaccinating a population, we have the hope of actually eradicating some diseases entirely. No vaccine is 100 percent effective; the more animals who have immunity and the fewer infections that occur, the less the chance that any one pet will contact the microorganism.

What do we currently know regarding how frequently vaccines should be given to pets?

Much research has been done into what is called the duration of immunity after vaccination. Though we do have quite a bit of data on this question, at this point we are still far from having all the answers. There are a number of obstacles to be overcome in trying to obtain definitive information:

- We must consider animal welfare. To accurately evaluate how long an animal is protected after being given a particular vaccine requires vaccinating test animals, keeping them in relative isolation (to reduce other factors that could influence the results, such as unintended exposure to the infectious organism), and then attempting to infect them periodically. An unvaccinated group of animals is kept and actually infected as a comparison. Although vaccine manufacturers do indeed carry out this sort of testing on dogs and cats, the more animals who are used and the longer they are kept in this manner, the more concerns arise.

  When pet vaccines were given annually, manufacturers only needed to demonstrate that resulting immunity lasted for at least a year. Now, in order to investigate how many years immunity actually lasts after various vaccines, long-term studies are required, and the welfare of the animals involved becomes even more of an issue.

- Another limitation of such experimental studies is that they are performed under artificial conditions. A vaccinated pet who is exposed to a disease naturally and an isolated animal living in a laboratory may not be affected in the same way.

- Several studies have measured antibodies against various diseases in pets who have been previously vaccinated. This method is less harmful to animals, but there are also drawbacks. For example, without actually trying to infect the animals, there is no way to know exactly what level of antibodies is required to protect against illness. In fact, we aren't even sure if any detectable antibody level is required, since the prepped immune system of a vaccinated pet may be able to quickly manufacture antibodies when required, and antibodies aren't the only component of immunity in any case. So we can use antibody levels as a clue to how long vaccinated animals are protected, but we can't rely on them to give us exact information.

Studies have shown that many (but not all) dogs and cats have measurable antibodies against certain viral infections for several years after vaccination. This is not true of every infection (for some, the antibodies don't last as long, and for some we don't yet have this information), but it does seem to be the case for several of the viral illnesses we most commonly vaccinate against (such as canine distemper virus, canine parvovirus, feline panleukopenia virus, feline herpesvirus, and feline calicivirus). The number of years that these antibodies persist varies from animal to animal; one dog's antibody levels might drop three years after vaccination, while another dog may still have antibodies five or six years after vaccination. Based on this information, many in the veterinary profession are moving toward less frequent administration of certain viral vaccines, most commonly to an every-three-year schedule.

The situation is complicated by several factors. One is that antibody studies have found a small percentage of vaccinated dogs and cats who did not have good antibody levels against these viruses, in some cases even when the interval since vaccination was not more than a year. Antibodies did not persist for the same period of time in different animals; in some pets they lasted for many years, and in others they faded more quickly. Additionally, there are many brands and types of vaccines. Data from one vaccine do not necessarily apply to other types of vaccine for the same illness. These kinds of issues make it difficult for veterinarians to say with confidence that vaccination intervals for every pet can be safely extended beyond a year. Some pets may not be adequately protected, even if most are.

It's important to understand that the duration of immunity provided by vaccines is extremely variable depending on the type of vaccine and the disease involved. Although traditional annual vaccination is rightly being reconsidered, a more scientific approach will result not only in some vaccines being given less often, but perhaps in some actually being administered more frequently to pets at risk. Particularly for certain bacterial infections, such as *Bordetella* (one component of kennel cough) and leptospirosis (an infection causing liver and kidney damage), vaccine-stimulated immunity is only short-term. You may have read sweeping proclamations stating that animals receive lifetime immunity from initial

vaccinations and that all boosters are unnecessary, but these pronounce-
ments do not take this sort of information into account. Some vaccines still
must be given at least yearly to provide protection.

Why can't we just measure antibody levels to see whether a pet needs booster vaccines?

It's possible that, for certain illnesses, we can indeed use blood tests
that measure antibody levels to determine whether an individual pet needs
booster vaccines. In fact, these tests are available for some pet diseases and
already in use by many veterinarians (such tests are also used in humans
for some situations). The problem is, we don't know exactly what antibody levels are protective against various infections (although we can
make educated guesses), and in fact we aren't even sure if measurable antibodies are necessary for good immunity. And for some diseases, because
of the way the infecting organism enters the body, the presence of antibodies on a blood test doesn't necessarily indicate adequate immunity. Additionally, laboratory tests cost more than vaccines, and not everyone would
be willing or able to perform periodic blood work on their pets. Many people would rather pay a smaller amount for a potentially unnecessary vaccine than spend more on a blood test that may indicate their pet needs the
vaccine anyway.

It all seems so complicated and confusing!

In some ways, it is. Although it's a good thing that the traditional
yearly vaccine intervals have been questioned, and that we're refining vaccine protocols to be as safe as possible while still effective, there aren't any
simple answers. The truth is that vaccine regimens really need to be tailored to the individual animal, based on lifestyle and environment as well
as owner preferences. Once you start doing that, things do get a lot more
complicated.

So what should I do about my pet's vaccines?

Your pet's personalized vaccine protocol must be designed by you
and a trusted veterinarian. To undertake this in an informed manner, you
should learn about the infectious illnesses affecting dogs and cats for
which vaccines are currently available. There is a lot of advice floating

around, on the Internet and from other sources, some baseless and much of it conflicting. I have seen completely false information presented as fact on the Internet, sometimes based on data that have been misinterpreted or exaggerated.

Without some understanding of how vaccines work and what their realistic risks and benefits are, along with knowledge about the relevant infectious diseases, there is no way for you to accurately judge the information that bombards you. By becoming educated in these matters, you can protect yourself and your pet from questionable advice no matter what the source.

Veterinary task forces have been formed to compile the most recent findings regarding vaccines and infectious diseases, and make up-to-date recommendations regarding immunization protocols. Based on the most current data, vaccines are periodically sorted into three categories: core (vaccines that every dog or cat should have), noncore (vaccines that are optional based on lifestyle and other factors), and not recommended (those that are felt to be unnecessary or contraindicated). Vaccines designated core protect against highly infectious organisms that cause severe illness. The noncore vaccines are those that your own pet may or may not need, and I will talk about ways you can decide this. As I discuss each disease, I'll talk about which category the corresponding vaccine falls into.

Who are the veterinary vaccine task forces? Can I trust them?

The American Association of Feline Practitioners, the veterinary organization devoted to improving the health and well-being of cats, has formed a Feline Vaccine Advisory Panel to develop and publish comprehensive recommendations. The most recent report can be viewed at www.aafponline.org. For dogs, the American Animal Hospital Association's Canine Vaccine Task Force has formulated the Canine Vaccination Guidelines; the newest version is available at www.aahanet.org, under "Resources." The members of these groups have meticulously reviewed the most current findings, in some cases themselves performing relevant studies. These veterinarians are highly regarded members of the profession and authorities in the field. I think that if you take the time to read one or both reports, you will find them quite thorough and objective. Although they are written for medical professionals, these reports are great resources for concerned pet owners who really want to educate themselves in this area.

What are the infectious diseases of dogs and cats for which vaccines are available?

Below is a list of illnesses against which we are currently able to vaccinate pets. Included is the task force categorization of each vaccine (core, noncore/optional, or not generally recommended). As you read through the information, make note of which vaccines seem appropriate for your pet on the checklist at the end of the chapter, and you will be well on your way to creating a personalized vaccination protocol for your dog or cat.

DOGS

Canine Parvovirus

The disease caused by this virus is often referred to simply as parvo. The virus attacks the lining of the intestines as well as the bone marrow. Due to severe intestinal damage, dogs with parvo will have diarrhea (often bloody) as well as vomiting. Because blood cells are produced in the bone marrow, the dogs will often have a very low white blood cell count. Dogs infected with parvovirus are extremely ill, usually requiring intensive care for a number of days. Even with treatment, the disease may be fatal, especially in puppies and certain dog breeds, including rottweilers, Doberman pinschers, and American pit bull terriers, who seem to be more susceptible.

Vaccine category: Core. This virus is highly infectious and can live for many months in the environment, so dogs are extremely likely to be ex-

---

Canine and Feline Parvoviruses

Feline panleukopenia is a severe illness in cats very similar to canine parvo. The two infections are caused by viruses from the same family, the parvoviruses (other species have their own parvoviruses as well). It is thought that the canine virus may have arisen from the feline version just a few decades ago. A little-known fact is that the canine parvovirus has now developed the ability to also infect cats. The feline panleukopenia vaccine may offer some protection, but a vaccine may need to be created to keep cats safe from this new threat.

posed. Even an indoor dog is at risk; the virus could be tracked into the home on shoes, for example.

Canine Distemper Virus

Canine distemper is an extremely serious viral illness in dogs and can cause many different symptoms including vomiting, diarrhea, respiratory issues, and neurological problems such as seizures. It has the highest fatality rate of any viral illness of dogs except for rabies. The name *distemper* can cause confusion because feline panleukopenia, which is caused by a parvovirus, is sometimes referred to as feline distemper, so canine and feline distemper are completely unrelated diseases caused by different families of viruses.

Vaccine category: Core. Canine distemper is highly infectious and causes severe illness. Some dogs who survive infection never fully recover; for example, permanent neurological damage may occur.

Canine Adenovirus

Dogs can be affected by two different adenoviruses, type 1 and type 2. Canine adenovirus type 1 affects the liver; this condition is called infectious canine hepatitis. Canine adenovirus type 2 is one of the organisms that can cause kennel cough, an infectious respiratory disease of dogs. Because vaccination against adenovirus type 2 will protect dogs against both types, and the type 1 vaccine has been associated with an immune reaction causing eye problems, dogs are generally vaccinated only against type 2.

Vaccine category: Core. This vaccine protects against both infectious canine hepatitis and kennel cough due to adenovirus. In general, vaccination against organisms causing kennel cough is considered optional depending on the dog's lifestyle: Dogs who are boarded or groomed, or go to day care, shows, or other environments with multiple dogs, are those who most need protection against kennel cough. The other vaccines protecting against kennel cough (the parainfluenza and *Bordetella* vaccines—see next page) are therefore designated as noncore. The adenovirus 2 vaccine is considered core because even though the number of cases of canine infectious hepatitis has decreased over the past few decades (likely thanks to vaccination programs), there is concern that this serious disease could once again become common if adequate vaccination does not continue.

Rabies Virus

Rabies is a virus that can infect all warm-blooded animals, including dogs, cats, and humans. The disease is almost always fatal. Infection is through saliva, most commonly via a bite wound. Canine symptoms are mainly neurological, including behavior changes, salivation, difficulty swallowing, hyperexcitability, seizures, and paralysis. Rabies vaccination of dogs is the law, with all states requiring an initial booster one year after the first vaccine. Many states then require boosters at three-year intervals, although some require more frequent vaccination.

Vaccine category: Core. Due to the fact that rabies vaccination is required by law, that infection is fatal in virtually all cases, and that there is a potential for transmission to humans, this is a core vaccine for both dogs and cats.

Canine Parainfluenza Virus

Canine parainfluenza (not to be confused with canine influenza) is another one of the organisms that can cause kennel cough in dogs. Symptoms of this disease include coughing that can last for weeks or even months and nasal discharge.

Vaccine category: Noncore (optional). Dogs who are frequently in contact with other dogs, such as those who are boarded, groomed, or go to day care or dog shows, should be vaccinated against parainfluenza and the other organisms that can contribute to kennel cough.

Bordetella bronchiseptica

Bordetella bronchiseptica is a bacterial organism that can cause kennel cough in dogs as well as upper respiratory infections or pneumonia in cats and other species. This infection can be transmitted between dogs and cats and can also affect humans. Like other sources of kennel cough, *Bordetella* infection is most likely in dogs who are often exposed to other dogs.

Vaccine category: Noncore (optional).

Borrelia burgdorferi (Lyme Disease)

The organism that causes Lyme disease is a spirochete—a kind of coiled bacteria. The disease is transmitted to dogs (and humans) via tick bites, most commonly by tiny deer ticks. Dogs can develop antibodies to Lyme disease from exposure to the organism with or without subsequent illness, or from vaccination, so a positive antibody test does not mean that a dog actually has Lyme disease. Dogs who do develop Lyme disease may have symptoms of arthritis (inflamed joints), and in some cases can develop heart or kidney disease or neurological problems. Prevention of tick bites is essential in protecting dogs from this infection, and there are excellent products available for this purpose, although none is foolproof.

Vaccine category: Noncore (optional). Lyme disease occurs throughout the United States, but it is much more prevalent in some areas (the website www.cdc.gov of the Centers for Disease Control and Prevention has helpful maps showing the incidence of Lyme disease around the United States). Lifestyle also affects the relative risk for this infection: Some dogs, such as those who live in or visit the countryside, are much more likely than others to be exposed to deer ticks. Preventive products against ticks, and owner vigilance regarding daily "tick checks" of the dog's body, go a long way toward preventing Lyme disease and other tick-borne diseases, although they are not a guarantee.

The decision whether or not to vaccinate against Lyme disease depends on a number of factors that vary widely among individual dogs. A dog who lives in the city and is carried about by her owner is obviously at low risk for the disease; a dog who runs loose in the woods of Connecticut is clearly at much higher risk. However, many dogs fall somewhere in between—suburban dogs, dogs who spend occasional weekends in the country, and country dogs who live in areas where the disease is uncommon. There are also other variables. A small dog with a short, white coat will be much easier to check for ticks than a large, long-haired dog with dark coloring.

In making this decision for your dog, you must consider all the issues that affect your dog's risk of becoming infected, such as the prevalence of Lyme disease in the area, your dog's lifestyle, the effectiveness of the tick-preventive products that you use, and your ability to thoroughly check your dog for ticks on a daily basis. Additionally, antibodies to Lyme disease can be measured, and it is widely felt by veterinary infectious disease experts that vaccination is not useful in dogs who already have Lyme antibodies. You may want to have your dog tested before vaccinating, but keep in mind that a positive test does *not* mean that your dog has Lyme disease—only that he has been previously exposed to the organism or vaccinated.

Leptospirosis

Leptospirosis is the term used for infection by various spiral-shaped bacteria that belong to a genus named *Leptospira.* The different members of this genus are called serovars, and several of them can cause illness in dogs. For example, dogs can be infected by the serovars *autumnalis, bratislava, canicola, grippotyphosa, icterohaemorrhagiae,* and *pomona,* among others. Many animals can be infected by leptospires, as can humans. Therefore, an infected dog could potentially transmit the disease to his owner or veterinary staff if proper precautions are not taken.

Dogs are infected through contact with the urine or tissue of an infected animal—another dog, a rat or other rodent, and others including raccoons, opossums, and skunks—or contact with water that has been contaminated by urine, such as a puddle or other moist area. Dogs in both rural and urban environments are at risk, since infected animals of various species can exist in both surroundings. The type of illness seen in dogs with leptospirosis varies somewhat depending on which serovar causes the infection, but the liver and kidneys are the organs most commonly affected, and jaundice (yellow eyes and skin) is often seen. The disease is treatable but can be fatal even with aggressive therapy.

Vaccine category: Noncore (optional). An individual dog's risk of infection is affected by factors such as the prevalence of leptospirosis in the area and the dog's lifestyle. Canine leptospirosis is on the rise, and illness caused by additional serovars is being seen. If leptospirosis occurs in your area, you should consider having your dog vaccinated unless she's one of those who never touch the ground. Since any puddle could be infectious, it is difficult to protect a dog against this disease without vaccination.

Various leptospirosis vaccines for dogs are available, some containing up to four different serovars. Dogs are only protected against the particular serovars in the vaccine they receive. You and your veterinarian can discuss which vaccine is most appropriate for your dog. Vaccination does not give dogs prolonged immunity against infection, and boosters must be given at least yearly, perhaps more often to dogs at high risk.

It is felt that some small-breed dogs (particularly pugs) and young puppies are prone to adverse reactions to leptospirosis vaccination, so puppies are not vaccinated until twelve weeks of age, and vaccination of small dogs is based on individual risk factors. Giving the leptospirosis vaccine on a different day from other vaccines may help reduce the chance of an adverse reaction; I recommend this for my patients if it's not too inconvenient for the dog's owner.

Giardiasis

Giardia is a microscopic intestinal parasite that can infect dogs, cats, humans, and other species. Different types of *Giardia* tend to infect specific mammalian species (the type most commonly infecting dogs, for example, is not the same as the one that usually infects humans), so the risk of human infection from an infected pet is thought to be relatively low, although it can occur. Dogs with giardiasis may have diarrhea (or more rarely vomiting), but often have no symptoms at all. Dogs generally become infected by ingesting *Giardia* cysts passed in another dog's stool, so those who are frequently in contact with other dogs, especially in dirty conditions, are most at risk. The cysts can survive for several months in water, so dogs (and others) can become infected by drinking contaminated water.

Vaccine category: Not recommended. The *Giardia* vaccine does not prevent infection with the parasite. It may prevent the dog from passing cysts in the stool.

Canine Coronavirus

This virus causes diarrhea in some dogs who become infected with it. Presently, there is debate as to the degree of illness caused by canine coronavirus and the usefulness of the vaccine in preventing dogs from getting sick. It has been difficult to determine the duration of immunity provided by this vaccine, for example, because the virus does not reliably cause illness even in unvaccinated dogs. There have been some recent reports in Europe of respiratory disease in dogs caused by a coronavirus.

Vaccine category: Not recommended. Many veterinary infectious disease experts are currently unconvinced that this virus causes significant problems for dogs, and thus do not feel vaccination is warranted. Veterinarians and dog owners should remain alert to changes in this situation, however.

Other Vaccines

New vaccines for dogs have recently been developed. A rattlesnake vaccine (*Crotalus atrox* toxoid or CAT) is intended to protect dogs who might suffer rattlesnake bites; this preps their immune system so that antibodies to the snake venom will help neutralize the toxic effects when a bite occurs. Another new product, the *Porphyromonas* vaccine, is designed to help prevent periodontal disease in dogs by immunizing them against three of the organisms that are suspected to contribute to this problem.

CATS

Feline Panleukopenia

Feline panleukopenia, also called feline distemper, is caused by infection with a type of virus called a parvovirus. A closely related virus affects dogs, causing the disease commonly known as canine parvo. From the Greek words for "all" (*pan*), "white" (*leuko*), and "decrease in" (*penia*), the name *panleukopenia* refers to the fact that this virus attacks the bone marrow of infected cats, leading to a very low white blood cell count. The virus also attacks the intestines, causing severe vomiting and diarrhea that may be bloody. If a pregnant cat becomes infected, the virus can damage the developing kittens' brains; brain damage can also occur if kittens are infected during the first few weeks of life.

Panleukopenia is a devastating disease, causing severe illness and often death, especially in young kittens. It is highly infectious, and unfortunately the virus can survive for up to a year in the environment, so cats can be infected by contact with any surface or item that another infected cat has touched, even long before. The virus can be carried into the home on shoes or other objects, so vaccination is essential even for indoor cats.

Vaccine category: Core. Due to the grave nature of this disease, and the fact that it is extremely infectious, all cats should be well vaccinated against panleukopenia. Canine parvovirus can also infect cats and cause illness; the panleukopenia vaccine may offer cats some protection against this related virus.

Feline Herpesvirus

Feline herpesvirus is one of several viruses that cause respiratory infections in cats. Disease caused by herpes in cats can range from mild to severe; symptoms include fever, sneezing, nasal discharge, corneal ulcers (defects on the surface of the eye), tracheitis (inflamed windpipe), pneumonia, and even skin conditions. Infected cats often stop eating, sometimes for long periods necessitating feeding tube placement, and due to corneal damage can lose vision in affected eyes. Some cats develop permanent nasal and sinus conditions. Like humans with herpes, infected cats harbor the virus forever, and can redevelop illness during times of stress or sickness, or if they receive corticosteroids (see chapter 7).

Vaccination against feline herpesvirus does not completely prevent infection (vaccines for some diseases can avert infections entirely), but it does lessen the severity and duration of illness. A vaccinated cat who is exposed to the virus may exhibit no symptoms, for example, or may have a few days of sneezing rather than becoming seriously ill.

Vaccine category: Core. Due to the highly infectious nature of feline herpesvirus and the severity of illness that can occur, including possible blindness and even death, this vaccine is recommended for all cats.

Feline Calicivirus

Calicivirus is another virus causing respiratory infections in cats. Symptoms of calicivirus infection include fever, sneezing, and nasal discharge, as well as pneumonia, oral ulcerations (open sores in the mouth), and swollen, painful joints. Some cats who have been infected with calicivirus become carriers and are infectious to other cats for months or years. Recently, more aggressive strains of feline calicivirus have emerged that cause severe symptoms including ulceration of various areas of the body, and are fatal in approximately 50 percent of affected cats. These dangerous strains seem to occur most frequently in living situations with large groups of cats, such as breeding colonies, boarding kennels, and shelters.

Like the herpesvirus vaccine, the calicivirus vaccine does not prevent infection or stop a cat from becoming a carrier, but instead protects exposed cats from the development of illness. Since there are multiple strains of feline calicivirus, the degree of protection provided by vaccination will vary depending on which strain a particular cat is exposed to. Vaccines may contain several viral strains for this reason.

Vaccine category: Core. Feline calici is easily transmitted between cats, is widespread, and can cause severe disease, so vaccination is recommended for all cats.

Rabies Virus

As described in the canine section above, rabies virus can infect all warm-blooded animals, including cats, dogs, and humans. The disease is generally fatal. Infection is through saliva, most commonly via bite wounds. In the United States, bats are the most common source of human rabies infection. Cases of feline rabies occur every year, however, and cats are more frequently diagnosed with rabies than dogs in this country. Cats with rabies develop neurological symptoms, and may hide or become more aggressive.

Most states legally require cats to be vaccinated. Some states allow boosters to be given every three years after the first yearly booster; others require more frequent vaccination, although this is generally felt by veterinary experts to be medically unnecessary.

The situation is complicated by the fact that feline rabies vaccination has been associated with the development of malignant tumors called fibrosarcomas in a low percentage of vaccinated cats (somewhere between one in one thousand and one in ten thousand vaccinated cats, although it is hard to say for sure since not all cases are reported). There has been much investigation into the reason for this, and the prevailing theory is that substances in the vaccines called adjuvants (agents used to stimulate an immune response to the vaccine), particularly aluminum, are likely the cause. Adjuvants cause an inflammatory reaction in the location where the vaccine is injected, and this inflammation is thought to eventually lead to tumor formation.

In response to this theory, new rabies vaccines have been developed that do not contain adjuvants. In feline studies, these nonadjuvanted vaccines don't appear to cause any more inflammation than an injection of plain saline. When we discussed the various types of vaccines in the beginning of the chapter, I mentioned recombinant vaccines, in which a virus that is harmless to the vaccinated animal is used to carry genes from the more harmful virus. A recombinant feline rabies vaccine that does not contain adjuvants and uses a virus called canarypox to carry genes from the rabies virus is now available. I use this rabies vaccine in my feline patients; you can discuss with your own veterinarian which vaccine your cat should receive. Unfortunately, the canarypox vaccine has not yet been legally approved to be used only every three years; cats must receive yearly boosters to comply with the law. Hopefully, this situation will change.

Additionally, it is now recommended that feline rabies vaccines be injected on the lower part of the right hind leg. If all veterinarians comply with this, it will be easier for the profession to determine how many cats develop fibrosarcomas secondary to rabies vaccination (fibrosarcomas can occur spontaneously, unrelated to vaccination, so it is sometimes difficult to determine whether vaccination played a role in tumor formation in a particular cat). And although this may sound grim, cats who develop tumors on the lower leg can often be cured by amputation; cats who were vaccinated on the back, as was done previously, had tumors that could not be surgically removed because of the difficult location. Hopefully, the canarypox vaccine will indeed prove to be safer for cats than rabies vaccines containing adjuvants.

Vaccine category: Core. Because of the fatal nature of rabies infection, and the fact that the disease can be transmitted to humans, rabies is considered a core vaccine. Some owners of indoor cats prefer not to vaccinate their cats against rabies; they are concerned about the possibility of a tumor, and feel that a cat who never goes outside is unlikely to be exposed (although it is important to keep in mind that bats are the most frequently infected species in this country and are known to get into homes). Veterinarians are in a difficult position, as rabies vaccination is generally required by law, and we know that even indoor cats sometimes get out. Owners of unvaccinated cats who are bitten by another animal or who bite a person can have legal difficulties, and it is our responsibility to convey all of this information to cat owners.

Feline Leukemia Virus

The name of this virus is often very confusing to people. Most people know that leukemia is a kind of cancer (bone marrow cancer), and so it seems as though a cat with feline leukemia must have cancer. In fact, the feline leukemia virus (abbreviated FeLV) is named in this way because one of the possible results of infection is the development of cancer, most commonly a kind called lymphoma. FeLV is a type of virus called a retrovirus; human immunodeficiency virus (HIV) and feline immunodeficiency virus (FIV) are also retroviruses. Cats who are exposed to FeLV may not become infected if their immune system is able to conquer the virus, but some cats become persistently infected, and are referred to as being FeLV-positive.

Transmission of FeLV between cats, which most commonly occurs through saliva, requires close contact such as grooming each other or sharing of food and water bowls. The virus can be passed from the mother cat to her kittens in the uterus, or through the milk. It can also be passed to a cat who is transfused with blood from an infected cat, so it's essential that feline blood donors be properly screened. Adult cats are much more resistant to infection than kittens, who are very vulnerable. Consequences of infection with FeLV include immunodeficiency (poor immune system function), anemia, and development of cancer, particularly lymphoma.

Like some feline rabies vaccines, some types of FeLV vaccine have been associated with the development of a kind of tumor called a fibrosarcoma (see the discussion earlier in the section on feline rabies virus vaccination). It is thought that the adjuvants (substances used to stimulate the immune response to vaccination) in these FeLV vaccines cause an inflammatory response where they are injected, which later leads to tumor formation. To help us keep track of these cases, the veterinary profession has designated particular locations for each vaccine to be given. FeLV vaccines should be injected into the lower part of the left hind leg. As I noted regarding rabies vaccination, vaccination on the lower leg rather than the upper body also allows a better chance of surgical cure if a tumor should develop.

Vaccine category: Noncore (optional). Because FeLV is only transmitted from cat to cat through close contact, an indoor cat who is not exposed to other cats is not at risk. If all cats in a household have tested negative for FeLV, they remain completely indoors, and no new cats are introduced, the FeLV vaccine is unnecessary. Owners should consider vaccinating cats who go outdoors or who live with an FeLV-positive cat (although if there is an FeLV-positive cat in the home, this cat should be kept separate from the others if at all possible). All cats should be tested for FeLV; vaccination has no benefit for a cat who is already positive.

It is important for cat owners to realize that the FeLV vaccine is not 100 percent protective against infection. The best way to prevent your cat from becoming infected is to keep him indoors or allow him outdoors only when supervised, and to test any new cat you are taking into your home. For owners who plan to allow their cats to go outdoors but are reluctant to vaccinate because of concern about side effects, one possible strategy is to only vaccinate cats under one year of age, since kittens are much more vulnerable to infection with the FeLV virus than adults. Keep in mind that adult cats can also become infected, however, even though the likelihood is less.

Feline Immunodeficiency Virus (FIV)

FIV is a retrovirus, like feline leukemia virus and HIV in people. Although FIV causes decreased function of the infected cat's immune system, it does not seem to cause as much illness in cats as HIV does in humans, and FIV-positive cats may live without symptoms for years. Issues that may develop in infected cats include stomatitis (inflammation inside the mouth), cancers such as lymphoma, diarrhea, weight loss, neurological problems, decreased blood cell counts, infections, and inflammation inside the eyes.

FIV is frequently passed from cat to cat through bite wounds that occur during fights, so it is most commonly seen in adult male cats who go outdoors, particularly those who are not neutered. Although it can be passed from an infected mother cat to her kittens, this is not common, and a positive FIV test in a kitten may be caused not by true infection but by temporary antibodies from the mother's colostrum (the earliest milk). For this reason, FIV-positive kittens must always be retested when they are six months old, since these maternal antibodies are gone by this time.

Vaccine category: Noncore (optional). There are several issues with the FIV vaccine. One problem is that there are multiple strains of FIV, and vaccination does not protect against all strains. An even bigger concern arises from the fact that the blood test for FIV checks for antibodies against the virus, and vaccination also causes these antibodies to form. Right now it is impossible to tell if a positive test is due to infection or prior vaccination, and once a cat has been vaccinated, there is no way to know if she becomes infected later.

Owners of cats who go outdoors and fight, or of cats who live with another cat who is FIV-positive, may want to consider vaccination. If a cat is vaccinated for FIV, he should be microchipped and wear an ID tag; if the cat becomes lost and ends up in a shelter or with a new owner and is tested for FIV, he may be euthanized. The best way to protect cats from FIV is to keep them indoors, and/or to neuter male cats so they are less likely to roam and fight. Of course, there is no point in vaccinating a cat who is already positive. The current vaccine does contain adjuvant (see the earlier sections on feline rabies virus and FeLV vaccination).

Chlamydophila felis

Chlamydophila felis is a bacterial organism that causes conjunctivitis and mild sneezing in cats. There is some concern that this infection can be passed from cats to humans. Similar to vaccination against feline herpesvirus and feline calicivirus, vaccination against *C. felis* does not prevent infection but may lessen the severity of symptoms.

Vaccine category: Noncore (optional). Cats who live in multicat situations where *C. felis* infection has been a problem may benefit from vaccination.

Bordetella bronchiseptica

Bordetella, a bacterial organism causing respiratory disease, is one of the agents causing kennel cough in dogs, and can infect humans. It is now known that this organism can also cause illness in cats, including sneezing, discharge from the nose and eyes, coughing, and even pneumonia. It is more common in situations where there are multiple cats. Cats who appear to be healthy can be carriers, and vaccinated cats may also spread the organism.

Vaccine category: Noncore (optional). Much like the situation with canine kennel cough, vaccination of cats who will be exposed to many other cats may be helpful. Unlike dogs, most cats stay at home, so this mostly applies to cats in boarding kennels, breeding colonies, and shelters, particularly those in which *Bordetella* infection of cats is known to be an issue.

Feline Coronavirus

Feline coronavirus is a complex topic. This virus can cause fairly mild vomiting or diarrhea, but can also result in a devastating disease called feline infectious peritonitis (FIP). Cats with FIP may have a persistent high fever, and can accumulate fluid in their abdominal or chest cavities that often causes them to stop eating and have difficulty breathing. There is no known effective treatment. It is unclear what causes a particular cat to develop FIP when exposed to coronavirus; viral mutations or more aggressive strains may be responsible, and stress or immune suppression likely contributes. Cats in crowded conditions are more likely to develop FIP.

There is no accurate blood test for FIP, as most cats have antibodies to feline coronavirus. The usefulness and safety of the feline coronavirus vaccine has been questioned, and studies have had variable results. There is a possibility that vaccination might induce disease in some cats.

Vaccine category: Not recommended.

Giardiasis

As we discussed in the section regarding the canine vaccine, *Giardia* is a microscopic intestinal parasite that can infect cats, dogs, humans, and other species. Different types of *Giardia* tend to infect specific mammalian species. The type most commonly infecting cats, for example, is not the one that usually infects humans, although people can become infected from pets. *Giardia* organisms are generally transmitted through contact with the stool of an infected animal, sometimes on objects, or by drinking contaminated water.

Cats infected with *Giardia* may have diarrhea, or may have no signs at all. The vaccine does not prevent infection but is intended to reduce symptoms and the number of *Giardia* cysts in the stool. There is not yet enough evidence of the effectiveness of this vaccine to recommend it. In addition, there is concern that the vaccine causes severe inflammation where it is injected, and this type of reaction to other vaccines has been suspected to cause fibrosarcoma tumors.

Vaccine category: Not recommended.

I've heard that vaccines have a lot of side effects. Is that true?

Vaccines can cause several types of side effects. It's important to minimize the chance of this occurring by tailoring vaccine protocols to individual pets, although there is little doubt that the risks associated with not vaccinating are much higher than the chance of a severe vaccine reaction. In fact, our success in greatly decreasing the occurrence of fatal infectious illness in pets has created a situation in which many pet owners are more concerned about the possibility of side effects than the diseases themselves.

Some adverse reactions to vaccines are virtually immediate. In dogs, itching, hives, and swelling of the face are some of the common symptoms of this type of reaction. In cats, vomiting and diarrhea may occur. Animals having this type of vaccine reaction can develop potentially fatal shock, and rapid treatment is essential.

Vaccines have also been suspected of causing what are called immune-mediated diseases: illnesses caused by the animal's own immune system attacking some part of the body. This has not been definitely proven to occur in pets, although there have been studies that support this possibility. Certainly, it may be wise to avoid repeating vaccines that have been suspected to have caused immune-mediated disease in a particular animal, or to minimize the use of vaccines in any pet who has suffered from this type of condition.

As we discussed in the section on vaccines for cats, a kind of tumor called a fibrosarcoma has been linked to certain feline vaccines. Substances called adjuvants that are found in some vaccines are thought to be the culprits. Newer vaccines have been developed that are hoped to be less likely to cause these tumors; you can ask your veterinarian to use these nonadjuvanted vaccines for your cat if possible.

Studies have indicated that the chance of an animal having an adverse reaction to vaccination increases with the number of vaccines given simultaneously. This is particularly true in small dogs. For this reason, it may be advisable to spread vaccines out over time rather than give them all at one visit. When designing your pet's personalized vaccination protocol with your veterinarian, you can talk over this possibility.

Hopefully, you now feel much more knowledgeable about your pet's vaccinations. You can use this knowledge to work with your veterinarian in formulating the most suitable protocol for your pet, and to ensure that your pet receives only those vaccines that will be of most benefit to her.

YOUR DOG'S VACCINATIONS: WORKSHEET

As you read about each vaccine, make a check in the appropriate column indicating whether you feel your dog needs this vaccine (I have already checked the core vaccines for you). You can also make notes here as you read through the chapter about issues that seem pertinent to your pet. At your pet's checkup, you can go over this list and your notes with your veterinarian and design a personalized protocol for your dog together.

Canine Vaccine Checklist

Vaccine	My Dog Needs	My Dog Does Not Need
Parvovirus (core)	✔	☐
Distemper (core)	✔	☐
Adenovirus 2 (core)	✔	☐
Rabies (core)	✔	☐
Parainfluenza (noncore)	☐	☐
Bordetella (noncore)	☐	☐
Lyme disease (noncore)	☐	☐
Leptospirosis (noncore)	☐	☐
Giardiasis (NR*)	☐	☐
Coronavirus (NR*)	☐	☐
*NR = not generally recommended.		

Notes

_____

_____

_____

_____

_____

YOUR CAT'S VACCINATIONS: WORKSHEET

As you read about each vaccine, make a check in the appropriate column indicating whether you feel your cat needs this vaccine (I have already checked the core vaccines for you). You can also make notes here as you read through the chapter about issues that seem pertinent to your pet. At your pet's checkup, you can go over this list and your notes with your veterinarian and design a personalized protocol for your cat together.

Feline Vaccine Checklist

Vaccine	My Cat Needs	My Cat Does Not Need
Panleukopenia (core)	✔	☐
Herpesvirus (core)	✔	☐
Calicivirus (core)	✔	☐
Rabies (core)	✔	☐
Feline leukemia (noncore)	☐	☐
FIV (noncore)	☐	☐

Vaccine	My Cat Needs	My Cat Does Not Need
Chlamydophila (noncore)	☐	☐
Bordetella (noncore)	☐	☐
Coronavirus (NR*)	☐	☐
Giardiasis (NR*)	☐	☐
*NR = not generally recommended.		

Notes

_____

_____

_____

_____

_____

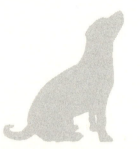

Dog Dermatologists and Cat Cardiologists:

When Your Pet Needs a Specialist

Think about all the different kinds of doctors you have seen during your life. When your teeth needed braces, you went to the orthodontist; when your skin was breaking out, you rushed to the dermatologist; and when your knee hurt from jogging, you saw an orthopedist. By specializing in particular fields, these doctors were able to take better care of you. In human medicine no one doctor is expected to be an expert at everything, and it is accepted that our health care often requires referral to one specialist or another.

The same is now true in veterinary medicine. There are veterinarians who provide general health care, and there are also many types of specialists who have advanced knowledge and experience in specific areas. To be sure your pet receives the best treatment, it's good to understand what the various veterinary specialists do and when your pet should see one. Knowing about the kinds of specialists that are available will help you to protect your pet when problems crop up.

What does it mean to be a specialist?

I have met many pet owners who thought their pet was seeing a specialist when in fact this wasn't the case. So this won't happen to you and your pet, you should know how to tell if a veterinarian is a true specialist. This title may only be applied to veterinarians who are board-certified by a veterinary specialty organization that is recognized by the American Veterinary Medical Association (AVMA). Specialists receive formal training in their chosen fields, usually through residency programs, and must complete a lengthy certification process.

For example, let's look at what is required to become an internal medicine specialist, also called an internist, for dogs and cats. After graduating from veterinary school, the next step is a one-year internship. Then the aspiring internist must spend several years completing a residency program that conforms to strict guidelines established by the American College of Veterinary Internal Medicine (ACVIM). The veterinarian must publish research or a case report in a respected medical journal, provide character references from associates, and pass two rigorous internal medicine examinations. Only then can the veterinarian become board-certified in small-animal internal medicine and use the title of veterinary internal medicine specialist.

All the veterinary specialties have similarly stringent requirements for board certification. This helps ensure that specialists in the various fields will be highly trained and qualified. By contrast, veterinarians cannot call themselves specialists simply because they are interested in a particular area, or because they limit their practice to an area. For example, pet owners may have the impression that a veterinarian is a specialist in a certain breed of dog or cat—but actually there is no such thing as a breed specialist. It's important for the term *specialist* to be used properly so that pet owners can be assured that anyone using this title has truly received advanced training and has been formally tested and certified.

Owners will sometimes mistakenly assume that anyone doing an advanced procedure, such as an ultrasound, must be a specialist. Although specialists are indeed trained to perform the procedures used in their field, this area of veterinary medicine is not regulated, and any veterinarian can offer to do a procedure regardless of training or experience. In chapter 5, there is information for you concerning which specialists have the most knowledge about performing particular procedures.

How can I tell if a veterinarian is really a specialist?

- Ask if he is board-certified, and in what area.

- Check for certain letters following his name. Board-certified specialists have designated titles that are given in the individual sections below.

- Contact the specialty's parent organization, or look on their website (see individual sections, or the list at the end of the chapter).

Where do specialists practice?

- Many practice in referral groups, where there are multiple types of specialists working together. At these facilities, your pet can benefit from a team approach. Suppose a pet needed major surgery but had a heart condition that could potentially increase the risks associated with anesthesia. A cardiologist at the practice would assess the pet's heart to determine the safest method of anesthesia, and then a surgeon would perform the operation. After the surgery, a critical care specialist would monitor the pet in the intensive care unit.

- Some specialists work in animal hospitals associated with veterinary schools, so check to see if there is a veterinary school in your area. In some cases, the cost of specialty care can be lower at a veterinary school than at a private practice.

- Other specialists practice in groups that include both general practitioners and specialists, or on their own.

- There are also traveling specialists, who visit various practices and perform procedures or consultations.

As an informed participant, you can help ensure that your pet gets the most advanced health care available. Learning about veterinary specialists is an important step in that process. By anticipating when your veterinarian might consider referring your pet to a specialist, or when you may want to request a referral or seek specialty care on your own, you can be a knowledgeable advocate for your pet.

What kinds of veterinary specialists are there, and what do they do?

Let's look at some of the types of specialists your pet might need and talk about what each one does. Because there are many fields of veterinary specialization, I'll focus on those you are most likely to encounter. You'll find a complete list of all the veterinary specialty organizations at the end of the chapter.

TIP To get more information about veterinary specialties, contact the American Board of Veterinary Specialties, which is part of the AVMA.

For each specialty discussed, I'll include:

- The specialty organization along with the website address. In addition to general information, these websites can help you find a specialist in your region.

- The specialist's title, indicated by initials that should appear after the specialist's name if she is board-certified. These initials generally start with *D* for "diplomate" (someone with a diploma in that area). For example, the initials *DACVIM* after my name mean that I am a diplomate of the American College of Veterinary Internal Medicine.

- Information about the specialty's role and when it might benefit your pet.

In the next chapter, I'll go into much more detail about some of the procedures that the various specialists perform.

TIP The American College of Veterinary Internal Medicine is the official organization of the veterinary specialties of small-animal internal medicine, large-animal internal medicine, cardiology, neurology, and oncology. Most of the other veterinary specialties have individual organizations.

Cardiology: American College of Veterinary Internal Medicine (www.acvim.org)

Title: DACVIM (Cardiology)

As you know from human medicine, cardiologists specialize in the diagnosis and treatment of heart disease. Veterinary cardiologists also often see patients who have pulmonary (lung) disease. The expertise of a cardiologist can make a real difference for animals with heart disease. Whenever I suspect heart disease in a patient, I have the pet evaluated by one of the cardiologists in my area. One of the primary diagnostic tools used by veterinary cardiologists is cardiac ultrasound; I'll talk more about this procedure in the next chapter.

There are two general categories of pets who may need a cardiologist: those with no symptoms in whom the veterinarian has found evidence of heart disease on a physical examination, and pets who are already sick from heart disease.

Heart Murmur, Gallop, or Arrhythmia in a Pet with No Symptoms

At your pet's checkup, your veterinarian may detect a heart murmur (abnormal heart sound), gallop rhythm (extra heart sound), or arrhythmia (abnormal heart rhythm). It is important not to ignore this finding. Although your pet may seem fine, these can all be a sign of a serious problem. Prompt diagnosis and treatment may improve both the length and the quality of an animal's life.

If an arrhythmia is detected, the cause should be promptly investigated. Since not all arrhythmias are caused by heart disease, your veterinarian may perform tests to look for other problems such as electrolyte imbalances, hormonal conditions, or even cancer. If these tests don't explain the arrhythmia, the pet should see a cardiologist as soon as possible.

Sometimes a gallop rhythm is heard in animals with heart disease, particularly cats. When we say that an animal has a gallop rhythm, we mean that there is an extra sound to the heartbeat. Normally there are two audible sounds (*lup-dup*); with a gallop there are three, so it sounds like a galloping horse. Gallop rhythms are almost always associated with heart disease and warrant evaluation by a cardiologist.

Causes of heart murmurs can range from mild to severe, and recommendations may differ based on your pet's age, species, breed, and the severity of the murmur. Let's talk more specifically about some of these groups.

Heart murmur in a puppy or kitten: Heart murmurs in young, growing animals can be what are called innocent or physiologic murmurs, which are harmless; or they can be caused by congenital heart disease, which can range from mild to severe. Physiologic murmurs are soft murmurs that generally disappear as the animal matures. Congenital heart disease can cause a loud or soft murmur, and requires consultation with a cardiologist. Some types of congenital heart disease require prompt intervention to prevent heart damage or death; early identification can be critical.

If your puppy or kitten has a soft heart murmur, your veterinarian may recommend that the murmur be reevaluated a short time later to see if it is gone. If not, or if it worsens, your veterinarian will likely refer you to a cardiologist. If the puppy or kitten has a loud murmur, you may be told to see a cardiologist immediately.

Heart murmur in an adult dog: Heart murmurs in adult dogs can be caused by leaky heart valves, abnormalities of the heart muscle, congenital heart disease, or noncardiac conditions such as anemia. If a murmur is detected in your adult dog, and no noncardiac cause is found, it is prudent to consult a cardiologist. If your dog has symptoms that may be related to heart disease, such as coughing, rapid breathing, exercise intolerance, or fainting, your veterinarian may recommend that you see a cardiologist right away. If your dog has a heart murmur but no symptoms, your veterinarian may recommend that you see a cardiologist at your convenience during the next few weeks or months.

Heart murmur or gallop in an adult cat: In cats, disease of the heart muscle (cardiomyopathy) is the most common type and can be quite serious. Unfortunately, not all cats with cardiomyopathy have a murmur, gallop, or arrhythmia to alert the veterinarian to a problem, although they may show signs such as panting after playing.

Cats may not have gradual symptoms of heart disease (as dogs frequently do, like coughing). Instead, they often have a sudden crisis. Many owners have no idea their cat has heart disease until she has an emergency, such as trouble breathing, collapse, or paralysis of a limb or limbs due to a blood clot caused by the diseased heart. The majority of cats with a heart murmur or gallop should see a cardiologist. Early identification and therapy may significantly improve your cat's length and quality of life.

Pets with Symptoms from Heart Disease

Pets with heart disease can have symptoms such as coughing or difficulty with exercise. Pets who are showing symptoms that may be caused by heart disease should see a cardiologist right away. There are several types of emergencies that can arise in a pet with heart disease.

Congestive heart failure: The most common emergency caused by heart disease in pets is congestive heart failure, in which fluid builds up in or around the lungs, or in the abdomen. Pets in congestive heart failure will usually have trouble breathing, which can be life threatening. Ideally, these patients should be hospitalized in a facility with twenty-four-hour monitoring and oxygen therapy.

Most animals in congestive heart failure receive similar therapy initially, including diuretics to remove the extra fluid from the body and oxygen to ease their breathing. The patient should see a cardiologist as soon as safely feasible. The cardiologist can identify the cause of the congestive heart failure and recommend more specific therapy to decrease the risk of it occurring again and improve the animal's length and quality of life. When I have a patient in congestive heart failure, I arrange for a cardiologist to come to the hospital as soon as possible. When there isn't a board-certified cardiologist who travels available, I have the owners bring the patient to the nearest cardiologist once their pet's condition is stable enough for a car ride.

Aortic thromboembolism: Cats with heart disease can have another type of crisis called an aortic thromboembolism. A thromboembolism is a blood clot. The aorta is the largest artery, carrying the blood supply from the heart to the rest of the body. Most often when a blood clot forms in the heart, it travels down the aorta and lodges at the point where the aorta forms a Y as it divides to supply blood to the two hind legs. Therefore, cats with this condition will often suddenly become paralyzed in the hind legs. Less commonly, one of the front legs is affected.

This condition, sometimes called a saddle thrombus, is very serious and can be accompanied by congestive heart failure as well. Your veterinarian will counsel you about your options; if you choose to attempt therapy, your cat will require immediate evaluation by a cardiologist for both a treatment plan and information about his prognosis.

Collapse or fainting: Pets with heart disease may also collapse or faint. These patients should see a cardiologist as soon as possible.

Dentistry: The American Veterinary Dental College (www.avdc.org)

Title: DAVDC

Dental disease is a common problem in pets. Imagine what would happen if you never brushed your teeth! In particular, many small breeds of dogs and brachycephalic (flat-faced) breeds of dogs and cats are genetically predisposed to dental disease. Unhealthy teeth and gums can lead to problems in other organs, so good oral health is essential for your pet's overall health.

Many general veterinarians treat routine dental disease in their practices. Owners are generally referred to a veterinary dentist if their pet has particularly severe oral or dental disease, or needs a specialized procedure. Some owners choose to utilize a veterinary dentist for all of their pet's oral health care because they feel more comfortable seeing a dental specialist.

Here are examples of some of the more common diseases I see in my patients that often require referral to a veterinary dentist:

- Feline odontoclastic resorptive lesions. This is a condition causing painful destruction of the teeth. It's a common dental problem in cats.

- Feline gingivostomatitis, a severe inflammation of the gums and mouth in cats.

- Fractured or traumatized teeth, including teeth that have been pushed out of the socket by an injury. When an animal has an injured tooth, such as a tooth that has broken, it must be addressed to avoid pain or infection. The owner may choose to try to save the tooth or may have the tooth extracted. If the owner elects to preserve the tooth, a veterinary dentist can perform procedures similar to those done in people with injured teeth, such as root canals.

- Jaw fractures and other facial fractures and injuries. Veterinary dentists can perform specialized procedures using dental acrylics to splint fractured jaws, and can also use these acrylics to help save teeth that have been pushed out of the socket.

- Diseases of the temporomandibular joint, which connects the jaw to the skull.

I also often suggest that patients who may need multiple teeth extracted see a veterinary dentist, whom I know will do the extractions very quickly and skillfully. Of course the animal will be under anesthesia, but I want this to be as brief as possible, and I know the dentist's experience and training mean the animal will likely feel less discomfort and have fewer complications later.

Dermatology: The American College of Veterinary Dermatology (www.acvd.org)

Title: DACVD

Just like dermatologists for people, veterinary dermatologists treat all kinds of skin conditions, which are a frequent issue in pets. Skin problems due to allergies are particularly common, so veterinary dermatologists treat many allergic patients.

Veterinarians will generally refer patients to a dermatologist when initial therapy has failed to solve the trouble, the condition is recurrent (keeps coming back), or the condition is severe or complex. For example, some animals with allergic skin disease are continually having problems. Animals with this condition can cause severe damage to their own skin because they are so itchy. Often a dermatologist is helpful in formulating the safest and most effective management plan, sometimes with the use of specialized allergy testing.

Believe it or not, skin disease can be life threatening, particularly when it's caused by the animal's own immune system. In autoimmune disease, of which there are several types, the body attacks itself. Autoimmune skin diseases can be extremely challenging to diagnose and treat, and dermatologists have advanced knowledge in this area.

Many skin conditions result in therapy with corticosteroids (cortisone-type medications) at some point. Although these drugs can be very helpful, they have significant side effects such as immune suppression, weight gain, and diabetes, and dermatologists can often offer alternatives. Their advanced training in this area helps them design treatment plans that eliminate or minimize the use of corticosteroids. As an internist who sees many patients with urinary tract infections, diabetes, and other medical issues resulting from the use of corticosteroids, I am especially appreciative of the skills of dermatologists.

Emergency and Critical Care: The American College of Veterinary Emergency and Critical Care (www.acvecc.org)

Title: DACVECC

Specialists in emergency and critical care, also called criticalists, focus on the treatment of life-threatening injuries and illnesses, and the care and monitoring of critical patients. They handle emergencies and lead intensive care unit (ICU) teams. They often work in emergency hospitals, referral centers, and veterinary schools.

TIP To prepare ahead for an emergency, the best plan is to locate a criticalist in your area if possible, and post the office location in your home. For example, you can check if any of the emergency hospitals in your area has a board-certified criticalist on staff. Similarly, if there is a veterinary referral group nearby, you can find out if they have a twenty-four-hour emergency service, and if they have an ICU run by one or more criticalists. If you live near a veterinary school, it may have an ICU with criticalists on staff.

On the ACVECC website, the following examples are listed of the types of patients who may benefit from a criticalist:

- Trauma patients, including those hit by cars, and those with bite, bullet, knife, or burn injuries.

- Any animal who is having trouble breathing.

- Animals who need a blood transfusion.

- Any patient in shock (signs of shock can include weakness, pale mucous membranes in the mouth, cold extremities, and an abnormal heart rate).

- Animals who are having trouble urinating, or are not producing urine.

- Dogs and cats who need specialized nutritional support because they are unwilling or unable to eat on their own.

- Animals for whom an abnormal heart rhythm is causing problems.

- Animals with life-threatening neurological disease such as coma or severe seizures that are not responding to medications.

- Patients who have had surgery and are not recovering well from anesthesia or are having trouble in the first few postoperative days.

"Hold on!" you might want to protest. "I thought you said that cardiologists treat abnormal heart rhythms. And doesn't an animal having seizures need a neurologist?" Criticalists treat patients who are in crisis, whatever the cause, and help to determine if the patient will need to see another type of specialist. They often work during evening, nighttime, or weekend hours when other specialists may not be available. Additionally, you can be reassured that any hospital at which the ICU is run by a board-certified criticalist is well prepared to deal with all kinds of emergencies.

Internal Medicine: The American College of Veterinary Internal Medicine (www.acvim.org)

Title: DACVIM

Internal medicine specialists are also called internists (not to be confused with interns, who are doctors performing their first year of postgraduate

Body Systems Included in Internal Medicine

- Nephrology: kidney disease.
- Urology: disease of the urinary tract.
- Gastroenterology: disease of the stomach and intestines.
- Hepatology: liver disease.
- Endocrinology: glandular and hormonal disease.
- Hematology: blood disorders.
- Pancreatic disease.
- Disease of other abdominal organs, such as the spleen and lymph nodes.
- Respiratory disease.
- Infectious disease.

training). Internists specialize in the diagnosis and treatment of diseases of the internal organs and systems. The sidebar lists the various body systems that fall under the category of internal medicine. Some internists may choose to focus on a particular area, especially those working in academic institutions or performing research. Most, like me, see a bit of everything.

Your veterinarian may refer your pet to an internist for help with the diagnosis and treatment of a problem in one of these areas, or for assistance in diagnosis if your pet has symptoms that have not yet been ascribed to a particular organ system. For example, if a pet has been losing weight or drinking more water and the cause is not clear, an internist can perform testing to help pinpoint the problem, and then give guidance as to the appropriate therapy. Below are some examples of the types of patients seen by internists.

Pets with abnormalities on a blood test, such as kidney or liver enzyme elevation, anemia, or electrolyte abnormalities: General veterinarians refer pets to internists for assistance in diagnosing the cause of these abnormalities and also for treatment recommendations. For an animal with a problem with the liver, kidneys, or another abdominal organ, the internist might perform an ultrasound exam, a test where sound waves are used to make a detailed image of internal structures. For an animal with anemia, the internist might use ultrasound to look for internal blood loss, or might take a small sample of bone marrow to see if red blood cells are being properly made by the body. In some cases, biopsy of an organ may be called for, and internists can often perform this noninvasively.

Pets with hormonal or glandular abnormalities, such as diabetes, Cushing's disease, thyroid problems, and others: Diabetes is a common condition in which the blood sugar is too high, generally requiring treatment with insulin injections. It is essential to closely control diabetes, and diabetic pets are often referred to an internist for consultation on the most effective type of insulin and assistance fine-tuning the insulin regimen. Cushing's disease is a condition where the body produces too much cortisol, a steroid hormone. This disease can be very challenging to diagnose and treat: It has multiple potential causes, and treatment can be fairly complex.

Pets who have a medical condition that is chronic (continuing or recurring), severe, or complex: For example, many pets will have a bout of vomiting or diarrhea a few times in their life, just as we all do. However, if a pet has vomiting or diarrhea that is severe or continues for weeks or months, and does not get better with standard therapy, that pet would need an internist to perform a consultation and possibly advanced testing such as an endoscopy. Similarly, a pet who develops a chronic cough or has repeated urinary tract infections may require an internist.

Pets with an internal medical condition requiring hospitalization in a facility with twenty-four-hour advanced care: Internists generally practice in hospitals that can provide intensive care for such conditions. For example, if a pet develops diabetic ketoacidosis (a situation in which a diabetic becomes critically ill due to toxins produced by the body when diabetes is not well controlled), the pet could be referred to an internist for hospitalization and aggressive treatment. A pet with severe anemia would be referred to an internist not only for diagnostics but also for hospitalization and a blood transfusion. Pets in kidney or liver failure likewise benefit from hospitalization under the care of an internist.

Pets whose symptoms are vague or perplexing: One of the jobs of internists is to solve medical puzzles using their knowledge, experience, and advanced diagnostic procedures. For example, pets with nonspecific symptoms such as lethargy, weakness, poor appetite, or weight loss might be referred to an internist. Internists use clues from the patient's history, physical exam, blood work, and other tests to narrow down the possible causes and arrive at a diagnosis.

As you can see, internal medicine is a very broad specialty, and internists see patients with a wide variety of conditions and symptoms.

Neurology: The American College of Veterinary Internal Medicine (www.acvim.org)

Title: DACVIM (Neurology)

Neurologists diagnose and treat disorders of the nervous system, including the brain, spinal cord, nerves, and muscles. Common examples seen in pets include epilepsy (seizures), slipped disks and other spinal problems, head or spinal injury, and meningitis. Neurologists also diagnose and help treat cancer of the nervous system, such as brain or spinal tumors. Many neurologists perform neurosurgery, such as spinal or brain surgery. Others work closely with surgeons who perform the operations recommended by the neurologist.

Pets displaying neurological symptoms—loss of balance, stumbling, pacing, bumping into things, disorientation, seizures, behavior changes—are referred to a neurologist for examination and advanced diagnostics such as a spinal tap or magnetic resonance imaging (MRI). These types of symptoms can be due to a variety of conditions, from infections to cancer, and it is crucial to pinpoint the cause promptly.

Pets can become suddenly weak or paralyzed due to a slipped disk (the proper name for this is a herniated disk) or another spinal problem. The general veterinarian will often refer them to a neurologist as an emergency, since it is crucial to relieve the pressure on the spinal cord as quickly as possible. If an animal with a herniated disk does not receive appropriate treatment rapidly enough, permanent paralysis can result. Surgery is often required. Disk problems are particularly common in certain dog breeds, such as dachshunds.

Veterinary neurologists often see pets with epilepsy that is difficult to control, and who continue to have seizures despite medication, or need dangerously high doses of medication. As an internist, I often see pets who have suffered liver damage due to phenobarbital, one of the medications used to treat animals with epilepsy. A neurologist can help prevent this type of side effect by suggesting a different medication or a personalized combination of several medications.

Oncology: The American College of Veterinary Internal Medicine (www.acvim.org)

Title: DACVIM (Oncology)

Oncologists specialize in the treatment of cancer. Just as for people, there have been many advances in this area for veterinary patients. Although treatment options for some types of cancer are limited, other cancers are relatively responsive to therapy. It is an individual decision for the pet owner whether or not to treat a pet's cancer, and how aggressively. An oncologist can offer not only a plan of therapy but also help the pet owner make decisions in an informed manner. When a pet has been diagnosed with cancer, owners are often confused and overwhelmed. The more educated owners are about their pets' condition, the more comfortable they will be with their decisions.

Pets may be referred to an oncologist when they have already been diagnosed with cancer, or when cancer is strongly suspected but more diagnostics are still needed. There are different ways to treat the various kinds of cancer, and oncologists sometimes work with other types of specialists to give their patients the best possible care.

One of the most common types of treatment is chemotherapy. This refers to the treatment of cancer with drugs, which are usually injected or given orally. When you hear the word *chemotherapy,* it may bring to mind all the side effects you have heard about in people, such as vomiting and hair loss. Although pets, too, can experience side effects, they are usually mild. Fortunately, most pets on chemotherapy do not lose their hair, and gastrointestinal side effects such as nausea and vomiting tend to be minimal or even nonexistent in dogs and cats. Many pets have no visible side effects at all. During the consultation, the oncologist will be able to give owners a reasonable idea of any side effects that are likely in their pet.

Oncologists may work with other specialists to provide the optimal plan for a particular animal. For example, the pet may need to see a surgeon for removal or biopsy of a tumor. Some kinds of cancer respond best to radiation therapy, which is performed by specialists in radiation oncology, a separate specialty from medical oncology. Working as a team, these specialists can approach the case as thoroughly as possible. An animal could have a tumor removed by a surgeon, and then have radiation therapy directed at the site to help prevent regrowth. Or an animal might have surgery followed by chemotherapy to target any cancer cells remaining in the body.

A helpful resource for owners of pets with cancer is www.vetcancer society.org. This website's information includes help with finding a specialist in your area.

Ophthalmology: The American College of Veterinary Ophthalmologists (www.acvo.org)

Title: DACVO

Veterinary ophthalmologists diagnose and treat diseases of the eye. They also perform surgery on the eyes, such as cataract removal, surgery to relieve glaucoma, and corneal surgery. Pets get many of the same eye problems as people, including dry eyes, glaucoma, cataracts, and corneal injuries, as well as a host of others.

Most eye problems in dogs are inherited, meaning they are due to the dog's genetics and seen most commonly in certain breeds. This is important because if you know that your dog is predisposed to a particular eye condition, you can monitor him for signs of a problem and seek immediate treatment if one arises. Since many eye problems can lead to blindness, time is of the essence if symptoms occur.

If you have a purebred dog, it is well worth investigating whether the breed has a tendency toward one or more ocular diseases; if so, you should monitor your pet closely or even consider preemptive evaluation by an ophthalmologist. For example, cocker spaniels are predisposed to several potentially blinding eye issues; if you have a cocker, you may want to consider having her eyes checked by an ophthalmologist periodically.

Cats are not as prone to inherited diseases of the eye, as very few pet cats are purebred. Although cats can develop all the same conditions as dogs, most eye problems in cats are caused by infections. These can be very serious as well.

Below are just a few examples of the types of conditions treated by veterinary ophthalmologists:

Dry eye: Properly called keratoconjunctivitis sicca (KCS), dry eye is a condition in which the eye does not produce enough tears. It is more common in certain dog breeds, such as shih tzus, and leads to blindness due to corneal damage if not treated properly. In pets with KCS, periodic monitoring by an ophthalmologist is prudent to ensure that everything possible is being done to preserve vision and minimize discomfort.

Glaucoma: In glaucoma, the pressure inside the eye is too high, causing pain and possible blindness. Certain breeds are also genetically predisposed to glaucoma, such as cocker spaniels. Any dog with glaucoma should be under the care of an ophthalmologist, as this disease is very challenging to treat and quite painful. The pressure inside the eye can rise very suddenly; if not treated immediately, this high pressure will cause permanent loss of vision. If your pet is suspected of having glaucoma, seek help from an ophthalmologist without delay.

Cataracts: Cataracts, which cause the lens of the eye to become opaque, can be inherited or caused by other diseases such as diabetes. Cataracts can often be removed surgically by ophthalmologists, restoring vision to animals unable to see. Pets with cataracts should be evaluated by an ophthalmologist, not only regarding the potential for surgery but also because cataracts can cause secondary problems in the eye that must be addressed to prevent damage and blindness.

Corneal ulcers: Erosions on the surface of the eye, corneal ulcers occur in both dogs and cats, but are more common in cats in whom they are often caused by viruses such as feline herpes. These viruses attack the cornea, sometimes leading to permanent damage or even blindness, especially if not treated promptly and appropriately. A cat with a corneal ulcer that does not heal readily with standard treatment should see an ophthalmologist for more specific care. Some corneal ulcers in cats and dogs require surgery to prevent the loss of the eye, so no time should be wasted if a pet has a nonhealing or deep corneal ulcer.

It is important not to ignore problems of the eye. If untreated for too long, they often lead to permanent damage and loss of vision. Untreated eye problems can also be very painful. Most eye problems are treatable if addressed promptly.

Radiation Therapy: The American College of Veterinary Radiology (www.acvr.org)

Title: DACVR (Radiation Oncology)

Radiation oncologists treat cancer using radiation therapy. This may be used as the main form of treatment, in conjunction with other types of therapy such as surgery or chemotherapy, or for relief of pain from tumors that cannot be removed.

Side effects of radiation therapy in animals are generally quite limited and manageable. The main side effect is dermatitis (inflamed skin) in the area receiving radiation. This is sometimes described as being similar to a sunburn. Veterinary patients usually do not experience vomiting or diarrhea from radiation therapy. Side effects will vary according to the area that is being treated and other factors, and the radiation oncologist will discuss this with the pet's owner before the decision is made to begin therapy.

Radiation oncologists generally work at veterinary schools or in referral groups. You may be referred to a radiation oncologist by your general veterinarian, by a medical oncologist, or by another specialist. For example, if a neurologist diagnoses a brain tumor in a pet, she may refer the patient to a radiation oncologist for treatment. Radiation oncologists often work closely with other specialists, such as medical oncologists, surgeons, and neurologists, to design and implement the most effective plan for the patient.

Although the field of veterinary radiation oncology is rapidly growing, there may not be a radiation therapy facility in your immediate area. This can be a hurdle, especially as some courses of therapy require treatments five days a week. Some owners choose to board their pets at the facility during the week, taking them home on weekends, or for the entire course of treatment, which is often about a month. Radiation oncologists have many patients who have traveled a long distance to receive treatment.

As mentioned in the section about oncologists, a helpful resource for owners of pets with cancer is www.vetcancersociety.org. This website's information includes help with finding a specialist in your area.

Radiology: The American College of Veterinary Radiology (www.acvr.org)

Title: DACVR (Radiology)

Veterinary radiologists have expertise in five areas of diagnostic imaging: radiographs (X-rays), ultrasound, computed tomography (CT), magnetic resonance imaging (MRI), and nuclear medicine (the use of radioactive substances to image the body). They use all these tools to help diagnose patients. There is more detailed information on these types of procedures in the next chapter.

Radiologists have advanced training in obtaining the highest-quality radiographs of a patient and interpreting the results. They are also proficient at performing ultrasound exams of various types. Although other specialists (particularly internists) often receive training in performing ultrasound exams, and most veterinarians perform and read radiographs in their practices, radiologists complete a three-year residency devoted to honing these skills. During this time, they also receive training in the use of computed tomography, magnetic resonance imaging, and diagnostic nuclear medicine.

Veterinary radiologists work in veterinary schools, referral groups, and other large hospitals; as consultants reading other veterinarians' radiographs; and as traveling specialists who visit various veterinary practices. Your pet may be referred directly to a radiologist for a procedure such as an ultrasound exam; if you are referred to another specialist at a referral group, that specialist may schedule an ultrasound exam or other test with the radiologist working at the facility.

Surgery: The American College of Veterinary Surgeons (www.acvs.org)

Title: DACVS

Veterinary patients are referred to a surgeon when they need advanced surgical procedures or for consultation and diagnosis when they have a problem for which surgeons have special training. For example, animals who have orthopedic symptoms such as limping or stiffness are often referred for evaluation to a surgeon who focuses on orthopedics. There are many kinds of operations for which an animal may be referred to a surgeon. They are generally divided into two areas: orthopedic surgeries and soft-tissue surgeries.

Some common examples of orthopedic surgeries include:

- Repair of torn cruciate ligaments in the knee.

- Surgery for luxating patellas (loose kneecaps).

- Hip replacement or other surgeries for animals with hip problems.

- Fracture repairs.

Soft-tissue surgeries that may require a specialist include:

- Abdominal exploratory surgery.

- Intestinal surgery.

- Surgery on one of the abdominal organs.

- Urinary bladder or gallbladder surgery.

- Thoracic (chest) surgery.

- Nasal or sinus surgery.

- Surgery on the larynx.

- Removal or biopsy of tumors in various locations.

- Wound repair.

Surgeons may work with other specialists at referral groups or veterinary schools or travel to various hospitals to perform consultations and operations.

You may be referred directly to a surgeon by your general veterinarian, or another specialist may determine that your pet needs surgery and have it performed by a surgeon who practices at the same facility. For example, imagine a pet who is referred to an internist for abnormal liver enzymes on a blood test. The internist performs an ultrasound exam and discovers that the gallbladder is diseased and needs to be removed. The internist may arrange for the surgery to be performed by a surgeon working at the same referral group.

Many surgeons work in facilities that have twenty-four-hour care, which is important for careful monitoring of patients who are recovering from surgery. Patients needing operations are often referred to surgeons to ensure that they receive proper postoperative care. During their residency training, surgeons learn not only about surgical techniques but also how to care for different types of postoperative patients and what types of complications are most likely to arise. Animals who have recently had major surgery should never be left alone overnight: They need to be monitored continuously and treated immediately not only for potential surgical complications but also for pain.

Behavior: American College of Veterinary Behaviorists (www.dacvb.org)

Title: DACVB

Behavior problems are of major concern for pet owners. Although certain behaviors may actually be "normal" in animals, they can be very difficult to live with. The truth is that behavior problems are one of the most life-threatening issues for pets, since they can lead to euthanasia, abandonment, or relinquishment to an animal shelter. Animal behavior is a growing and very necessary field; finding the right behaviorist can be as critical to the pet's health and welfare as any of the other veterinary specialties.

Common canine behavior problems include issues such as aggression toward people or other animals, destructiveness, fear of thunderstorms, or other fears, separation anxiety and other forms of anxiety, housebreaking issues, submissive urination, and excessive barking. Feline behavior problems include issues such as house soiling (urination or defecation in inappropriate areas), aggression, destructiveness, fear, or shyness.

The first thing you should do if your pet develops a behavior problem is consult with your veterinarian to make sure that the issue does not have an underlying medical cause. For example, inappropriate urination can be due to a urinary tract infection or bladder stone, inappropriate defecation can result from a gastrointestinal problem, and aggression may be due to a painful condition or a neurological problem.

Once your veterinarian determines that the problem is not medical, there are several places you can turn for help. Below are three different groups that may be helpful. The first group is the veterinary behavior specialty itself; the other two are nonveterinary groups that also focus on behavioral issues in pets.

Certified veterinary behaviorist: Veterinarians can become board-certified behaviorists who provide consultation on pet behavior issues and if necessary prescribe drugs to help modify behavior. To find one in your area, contact the American College of Veterinary Behaviorists. Since a fairly limited number of veterinarians belong to this specialty, there may not be a veterinary behaviorist in your area.

Certified applied animal behaviorist: These specialists can be veterinarians or nonveterinarians with doctorate (PhD) degrees. Applied animal behaviorists are certified by the Animal Behavior Society, which can be contacted to locate one in your area (www.animalbehavior.org). Nonveterinarians cannot prescribe drugs, but the behaviorist will work with your veterinarian, who can.

Certified pet dog trainer: For some behavior problems in dogs, you may find it helpful to work with a dog trainer. Or you may turn to a dog trainer if there isn't a certified veterinary behaviorist or certified applied animal behaviorist in your area. The Certification Council for Pet Dog Trainers (CCPDT) is the national organization that provides certification for dog trainers. The situation can be very confusing: Many schools offer certification for their specific dog-training courses, but the CCPDT is a national organization with standardized testing and monitored exams. Only candidates who pass this exam can use the title of certified pet dog trainer and include the letters *CPDT* after their names.

THE VETERINARY TEAM

These two stories illustrate how veterinary generalists and specialists can work together to help pets with health problems.

The Story of Sparkles

Maria's puppy Sparkles has been acting strangely. He gets very dizzy and tired after he eats, and sometimes acts like he can't see. She makes an appointment with her veterinarian. When she tells her veterinarian about Sparkles's symptoms, he is concerned that Sparkles may have a shunt. He explains that some animals are born with an abnormal blood vessel called a shunt that allows their blood to bypass the liver. This causes toxic substances to build up in the bloodstream and affect the brain, causing neurological symptoms.

Maria's veterinarian performs a special blood test used to diagnose shunts called a bile acids test, and the results are abnormal. He tells Maria that he wants Sparkles to have an ultrasound exam performed by a radiologist, so Maria brings Sparkles to the radiologist at the referral hospital in her area. The radiologist performs the ultrasound exam and tells Maria that she does see a shunt near Sparkles's liver. Maria's veterinarian and the radiologist both recommend that Sparkles have surgery to correct the shunt. Maria is referred to the surgeon who works in the same referral group as the radiologist.

The surgeon explains to Maria that there is some risk to performing the surgery, but in Sparkles's case the risk is much higher if the shunt is not repaired. Maria decides to go ahead. The surgeon sends Sparkles home on a special diet and several medications to stabilize him before the surgery is performed. On the day of the operation, Maria drops him off at the hospital, feeling very nervous. Later that afternoon, the surgeon calls Maria to tell her that the surgery to close the shunt was successful; Sparkles is out of anesthesia and groggy but awake.

Sparkles must be watched closely for the next few days, since there is a risk that he will develop seizures or other problems in the postoperative period. He will be in the ICU under the care of the criticalist for at least the first two days.

Sparkles does well over the next few days, and is discharged from the hospital with instructions to have his regular veterinarian perform a follow-up blood test in a month. Maria is given the name of the internist at the hospital where the surgery was performed, who can help fine-tune Sparkles's medication if necessary over the next few months and assist in treating the dog if further liver problems develop.

The Story of Mittens

Peter notices a lump on his cat Mittens's lower back. He takes her to his veterinarian, who is worried that it may be a tumor. The veterinarian performs a biopsy, and when the results come back she tells Peter that Mittens has a kind of tumor called a fibrosarcoma. She explains that in some cats, this kind of tumor may be caused by a rabies vaccine. She refers Peter and Mittens to an oncologist for advice.

The oncologist gives Peter a lot of information about Mittens's tumor. He explains that the most successful therapy for this kind of tumor seems to be a combination of surgery and radiation therapy. The surgery is intended to remove as much of the tumor as possible—hopefully all of it. He tells Peter that according to research, a successful surgery is very important with this kind of tumor. He recommends a surgical specialist for the procedure.

They also talk about radiation therapy. The oncologist explains that studies have shown that cats with this kind of tumor who have both radiation therapy and surgery tend to do best. The radiation therapy can be done before or after the surgery. In Mittens's case, he recommends they do the radiation therapy first, to shrink the tumor so the surgery will have a better chance of success. When Peter meets with the radiation oncologist, she describes the course of therapy. Mittens would receive radiation therapy five days a week for a month. Each session will only take a few minutes, but Peter needs to decide if he can handle this intensive schedule with all his other responsibilities. It's a big decision.

Peter goes home to think about it and talk it over with his family. They decide to go ahead with the radiation therapy and surgery. If they all pitch in and help transport Mittens back and forth, they can handle it for a month. Mittens starts radiation therapy the next week. She is annoyed by the traveling and looks funny with the shaved spot on her back, but she eats and purrs like always. It is a tough month, but it goes by quickly and Mittens seems to handle it fine. She has a bald spot on her back; the radiation oncologist says her hair will grow back, but probably in a different color.

The next step will be to schedule the operation with a surgeon.

Just as for your own health, specialists are an important component of your pet's medical care. In addition to the veterinary specialists I've described in detail, there are others working to keep pets and other animals healthy. Some of these specialists may help pets behind the scenes. For example, a veterinary anesthesiologist may help monitor your pet under anesthesia for a surgery or procedure. A veterinary pathologist examines biopsies and other laboratory tests so pets can be accurately diagnosed. If your pet eats something dangerous, you may call a poison control line and speak to a veterinary toxicologist.

Another type of veterinary specialist who can be very helpful to pet owners is a veterinary nutritionist. Nutritionists can advise on the best diet for a particular animal, and can also formulate balanced homemade diets for pets. Especially in the wake of the extensive pet food recall that occurred in the spring of 2007, many people are interested in feeding their pets homemade food. However, it is essential that a pet's diet be carefully balanced so that dangerous nutritional deficiencies or excesses do not occur. Nutritionists can offer general diets that are balanced for all healthy dogs or cats, or can create personalized diets for animals with medical conditions or food preferences. Websites that are staffed by board-certified nutritionists and offer these services include www.petdiets.com and www.balanceit.com.

If you think your pet may need a specialist, there are several ways to go about seeing one. Some specialists only see pets who have been referred by the general veterinarian. Your veterinarian may have already suggested that your pet see a specialist; if not, you can ask for a referral. Some specialists do not require a referral. Most veterinarians will be very supportive of your desire to seek assistance from a specialist, and the AVMA guidelines encourage timely referral. If your veterinarian discourages you from seeking specialized care for your pet, you should be concerned.

If you do decide to see a specialist, be sure to bring all your pet's medical records and copies of radiographs and other test results. This will make the appointment far more valuable for you and your pet, and may also save you money—if you don't bring your records, some tests may need to be repeated. Don't feed your pet for eight hours before the appointment in case the specialist chooses to perform a procedure the same day. The exception would be a pet who should not fast, such as a diabetic or a pet who is very small, young, or weak.

There are various means to find a specialist in your area. Often, your regular veterinarian will be able to recommend a specialist or referral group. You can also go to the specialty's website. Some list specialists geographically, or you can contact the organization and ask for the names of doctors in your area. If there is a veterinary school near you, there will be many specialists on staff. You can also search for members of a specialty on the Internet, or check your phone book for referral groups.

VETERINARY SPECIALISTS: THE FULL ROSTER

Below is a list of all of the veterinary specialties, along with the websites you can visit for more information.

- American Board of Veterinary Practitioners: www.abvp.com

- American Board of Veterinary Toxicology: www.abvt.org

- American College of Laboratory Animal Medicine: www.aclam.org

- American College of Poultry Veterinarians: www.acpv.info

- American College of Theriogenologists (reproductive medicine): www.theriogenology.org

- American College of Veterinary Anesthesiologists: www.acva.org

- American College of Veterinary Behaviorists: www.dacvb.org

- American College of Veterinary Clinical Pharmacology: www.acvcp.org

- American College of Veterinary Dermatology: www.acvd.org

- American College of Veterinary Emergency and Critical Care: www.acvecc.org

- American College of Veterinary Internal Medicine (internal medicine, cardiology, oncology, and neurology): www.acvim.org

- American College of Veterinary Microbiologists: www.vetmed.iastate.edu/acvm

- American College of Veterinary Nutrition (can help formulate balanced homemade diets): www.acvn.org

- American College of Veterinary Ophthalmologists: www.acvo.org

- American College of Veterinary Pathologists: www.acvp.org

- American College of Veterinary Preventive Medicine: www.acvpm.org

- American College of Veterinary Radiology: www.acvr.org
- American College of Veterinary Surgeons: www.acvs.org
- American College of Zoological Medicine: www.aczm.org
- American Veterinary Dental College: www.avdc.org

DOES MY PET NEED A SPECIALIST?: WORKSHEET

If the answer to any of the following questions is yes, your pet may need a specialist.

- Have your pet's symptoms been going on for a month or more despite treatment?
- Are your pet's symptoms recurring?
- Is your pet going downhill rapidly (experiencing worsening symptoms, losing weight, becoming weaker)?
- Is your pet's condition difficult to diagnose?
- Is your pet's condition difficult to control?
- Is your pet in pain despite treatment?
- Is your pet having side effects from his current treatment?
- Is your pet's condition critical?
- Does your pet need advanced diagnostics (ultrasound exam, echocardiogram, endoscopy, CT, MRI)? See chapter 5 for more details.
- Does your pet need major surgery?
- Does your pet have a heart murmur, heart arrhythmia, heart gallop, or congestive heart failure?
- Does your pet have cancer?
- Is your pet losing her vision or having eye discomfort?
- Does your pet have a chronic or painful condition in the mouth?
- Does your pet have an injured tooth you would like to save?

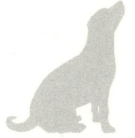

CHAPTER 5

CAT Scans and Dog Scans:

Advanced Technology for Your Pet

Remarkable advances have taken place in the medical technology available to doctors and veterinarians, including our ability to noninvasively diagnose and treat illness and injury. We are able to see inside our patients' bodies and image the organs and structures there with amazing detail. We can find abnormalities, take samples, and in some cases perform repairs without invasive surgery.

When I consider how fortunate my patients and I are to have the use of modern diagnostic tools, I can't help but compare myself with veterinarians who not so many years ago had only their senses and a scalpel to rely on. Now I can use an endoscope to remove a toy that is lodged in a puppy's stomach, or ultrasound to locate and biopsy an intestinal tumor. Only a few decades ago, these patients would have needed surgery.

As helpful as it is for human and animal patients, the proliferation of technology can be confusing to the pet owner. You may be familiar with some procedures from your own experiences, but unsure of how they will be used for your pet. Will he need to be sedated or anesthetized? How will this procedure help him? Is it dangerous? Which doctor is best qualified to perform it?

In this chapter, I'll talk about a number of procedures that are used in veterinary medicine today. For each one, I'll help you understand what it is and how it is done, why a pet would need it, and what the risks are. I will focus on the more specialized diagnostic procedures that may be unfamiliar to you.

I'll also talk about which type of specialist generally performs each of these procedures. Just as in human medicine, veterinary specialists in particular fields are trained in certain technologies, although for a few procedures there is some overlap. The situation is complicated by the fact that equipment for advanced procedures can be purchased and used by any licensed veterinarians, regardless of whether or not they are specialists in the field or have adequate training. No certification is required. Therefore, it is very important for pet owners to examine the qualifications of any doctor who may perform procedures on their pet. Only you can protect your pet by checking on this, so if a procedure is being recommended, be sure to ask about the credentials of whoever will be doing it.

I believe educated pet owners can play a vital role in their pet's health care. I have seen many owners help their ailing pets by arming themselves with knowledge and taking the initiative to demand the best care available. You can use the information in this chapter to better understand a procedure that has been recommended for your pet, and to be sure that the proper person is performing it. You can also use it as a guide to the types of advanced diagnostics that are available in veterinary medicine, and to when you might want to seek out one of these tools for your pet.

A note regarding risks: Please realize that the risks I have listed are general, and it is essential to discuss your own pet's particular situation with any doctor who will be performing a procedure. Any procedure requiring anesthesia carries anesthetic risks that vary with the overall health of the patient and the type of anesthesia used.

ULTRASOUND

Ultrasound scans, also called sonograms, use high-frequency sound waves to form images of tissues within the body. Ultrasound technology is similar to the sonar used by bats and by ships at sea. The sound waves are reflected by the patient's tissues, and these reflected sound waves are recorded and displayed as a visual image. This occurs in real time: The images are immediately displayed on a screen that looks like a television or computer monitor. Because of this, the doctor can form not only pictures of the organs and tissues but also observe certain things as they happen, such as blood flow, heartbeats, and other activity within the body.

In veterinary medicine, ultrasound is most commonly used to examine the abdominal organs and the heart, as well as other parts of the body like the thyroid and parathyroid glands, the testicles, and the eyes. Because ultrasound waves cannot pass through bone or air, the procedure is not generally used to look at the lungs. However, when a disease, such as a tumor or abscess, replaces air in a lung lobe, ultrasound may sometimes be used to examine that part of the lungs.

Abdominal Ultrasound

When would a pet need this?

Abdominal ultrasound is used when a veterinarian suspects an animal has disease in one of the organs or in the abdominal cavity itself. For example, the veterinarian may have discovered an abnormality on a blood test that indicates a problem with an organ such as the liver or kidneys, or he may feel something unusual in the abdomen on a physical examination.

He Ate *What*?

Ultrasound can be very useful to figure out why an animal is vomiting. When a dog or cat has been vomiting, one of the things veterinarians worry about is that she may have eaten something that is causing an intestinal obstruction. Animals eat all sorts of crazy things: toys, corncobs, rubber bands, shoes . . . you name it.

Although we cannot always see foreign objects within the intestinal tract using ultrasound, we are at least often able to determine that there is some type of obstruction. With the amazing machines used today, we can see something as small as a string that an animal has swallowed and that is tangled in the intestines. By confirming our suspicions quickly, we can rush the patient to surgery before it's too late.

The animal may have symptoms suggesting a problem in the abdomen, like vomiting or poor appetite.

Examples of organs that can be evaluated by this method include the liver, gallbladder, kidneys, spleen, urinary bladder, pancreas, adrenal glands, uterus, ovaries, and prostate gland. The gastrointestinal tract (stomach and intestines) can also be evaluated, although gas inside the GI tract may make it difficult to visualize some parts. (Remember, ultrasound cannot pass through air, and intestinal gas is air.)

When an animal has fluid in the abdominal cavity—as is seen in congestive heart failure, liver disease, or certain infections, or as a result of a ruptured organ—ultrasound is especially useful. The fluid in the abdominal cavity will obscure the detail of X-rays, but it will not impede ultrasound scans.

Who performs it?

- Radiologists receive the most training in performing ultrasound exams. If one is available in your area, a radiologist is an excellent choice.

- Internal medicine specialists receive ultrasound training during their residencies, and in addition have advanced knowledge of the diseases of the abdominal organs. They are skilled at interpreting the results of the ultrasound scan and making recommendations, whether they perform it or it's done by a radiologist.

Because anyone can buy an ultrasound machine, individuals who do not have sufficient training sometimes perform this procedure. There is a world of difference between a radiologist who completed an intensive three-year residency program and a doctor who took a weekend course or just bought a machine for his practice. Unfortunately, an unskilled ultrasound exam can do more harm than good, since inaccurate results may lead to incorrect diagnosis or treatment. Don't be afraid to ask the doctor who will be performing your pet's ultrasound exam how he received his training.

What are the risks?

Ultrasound scans pose no known risks. Because the procedure is generally painless, most animals will not need to be sedated. However, there are a few exceptions. If an animal has abdominal pain from the illness

Remote Ultrasound

An increasingly popular method in veterinary medicine is for someone at a practice to perform an ultrasound scan of the abdomen or heart, and then send pictures to a specialist (such as a radiologist, internist, or cardiologist) for interpretation. Although it may be convenient for veterinary practices, my concern with this method is that looking at a picture is not the same as actually performing a scan, particularly depending on the training of the individual and the quality of the images.

To closely examine the liver, for example, a specialist performing a scan will sweep through the whole organ several times, looking for any abnormalities. What happens instead with the remote method is that the specialist ends up interpreting a few pictures that may or may not include any abnormal areas. The specialist can only interpret the images that are given to her, and often she will feel uncomfortable about informing the practice if the images are of poor quality.

If a subtle abnormality such as an enlarged lymph node, localized intestinal thickening, or small lump in an organ is not noted and recorded, the specialist doing the interpretation will have no knowledge of its existence. Imagine if you were thinking of buying a house and could only see photos. If you wanted to know what the living room looked like and someone sent you a picture of just one corner, you would have no way of knowing that there was a crack in the plaster in the opposite corner and a water stain on the ceiling.

I believe this method should be reserved for situations when it is the only option—there is no specialist available to perform the scan. If there is a qualified specialist in the geographic area, the pet owner should be advised of this option.

being diagnosed, she may feel some discomfort from the pressure as the scan is performed, and sedation may be necessary. If an animal is very squirmy, frightened, or defensive, she may need to be sedated, since it is difficult to perform an accurate scan when a patient is panting, whining, struggling, or very tense. In these instances, the risks are those associated with sedation.

Heart Ultrasound (Echocardiogram)

When would a pet need this?

Echocardiograms are often recommended for pets who have heart murmurs, arrhythmias, or gallops (discussed in chapter 4); for pets who have developed congestive heart failure or are suspected of having tumors on or near the heart; and for some pets with heartworm infections.

Who performs it?

- Cardiologists complete a three-year residency devoted to studying the heart, performing echocardiograms and other cardiac procedures, and treating heart disease. They are also the most qualified to make recommendations based on the results. If there is a cardiologist in your area, this should without doubt be your first choice.

- If you cannot locate a cardiologist, your next choice would be radiologists and internal medicine specialists, who are often trained to perform echocardiograms. Before making an appointment with a particular doctor, make sure she performs echocardiograms—not all specialists in these fields do.

What are the risks?

There are no known risks to this procedure. If the pet requires sedation, the risks are those associated with the sedation.

Ultrasound Scan of Other Body Parts

When would a pet need this?

A pet may need an ultrasound exam of the chest cavity if he is suspected of having fluid, a tumor, or other abnormality such as an enlarged lymph node or abscess inside the chest. Ultrasound scan of the thyroid glands, parathyroid glands, or testicles may be recommended if these organs are enlarged or suspected of being diseased.

Who performs it?

Radiologists have the most training in these types of ultrasound scans; many internal medicine specialists are also trained in these areas.

What are the risks?

There are no known risks to these procedures. If the pet requires sedation, the risks are those associated with the sedation.

Ocular Ultrasound (Ultrasound of the Eye)

When would a pet need this?

Ultrasound is used to examine the eye when an abnormality prevents the ophthalmologist from performing a complete ophthalmic examination. Before performing cataract surgery, for example, the ophthalmologist must be sure the animal's retina is normal, yet the cataract may prevent full visualization of the retina at the back of the eye. Ultrasound can be used to make sure the retina is intact.

Ultrasound can also be used to examine the eye for foreign objects, evaluate the eye following trauma, investigate suspected tumors, and examine the area behind the eye.

Who performs it?

Radiologists. Some ophthalmologists are also trained to perform ocular ultrasound scans. It is generally an ophthalmologist who is recommending the scan and interpreting the results, so your pet's ophthalmologist will advise you on who should perform the procedure.

What are the risks?

Most animals do not require sedation for this procedure, which can generally be done with only topical anesthesia (numbing the surface of the eye with drops). Corneal irritation is a possibility, but precautions are usually taken to avoid this.

ENDOSCOPY

Endoscopy uses fiber optics (long strands of glass or other light-transmitting materials that are bundled together and encased in rigid or flexible scopes of various sizes) to examine various parts of the body. More recently, video endoscopy has been developed, using a tiny, optically sensitive computer chip at the tip of the scope. The appropriate scope for the particular procedure is inserted into the body through a natural opening or small incision, and the image from inside the body is displayed on a screen. Many scopes have slender channels that water, air, or suction is delivered through when needed to help the doctor see, and another channel for a biopsy instrument (armed with tiny jaws) that takes samples. These channels are also used for instruments that reach inside the body to remove objects or to perform other tasks.

In many ways performing an endoscopy, which involves the simultaneous manipulation of multiple knobs and buttons, is similar to playing a musical instrument. I first thought of this during my residency while watching a talented endoscopist in action. And similar to playing an instrument, endoscopy takes training and then lots of practice to master.

Upper and Lower Gastrointestinal Tract (Upper GI Endoscopy and Colonoscopy)

Endoscopy of the gastrointestinal tract allows examination inside the esophagus, stomach, and intestines. Many people are familiar with colonoscopy, which is endoscopy of the colon (large intestine). For this procedure, the large intestine is entered rectally. The patient's colon must be cleaned out before colonoscopy is performed, which involves the use of enemas, laxative-type solutions, or both. For upper GI endoscopy, the instrument is passed through the mouth, down the esophagus, into the stomach, and then into the small intestine. The only preparation generally required is an overnight fast. In this procedure, the endoscope can usually reach only the first section of the small intestine, called the duodenum.

Although the GI endoscopy isn't painful, it does require anesthesia; otherwise animals would never allow the procedure to be done! Anesthetizing an animal also makes it possible for the doctor to place a tube in the trachea (windpipe) to prevent material from the GI tract from entering the lungs. There is generally no discomfort after the procedure.

When would a pet need this?

Pets who have GI symptoms, such as vomiting, diarrhea, blood in their stool, poor appetite, or weight loss, may have endoscopy for examination and biopsy of the GI tract. Pets who have swallowed an object that becomes lodged in the esophagus or stomach may have the object removed by endoscopy rather than surgery, as long as the object is within reach of the endoscope. For pets who can't or won't eat on their own for a period of time, endoscopy can be used to place a small tube through the animal's side into the stomach, which is in some situations the best way for pet owners to feed and medicate their ill pets without a struggle. My tech-

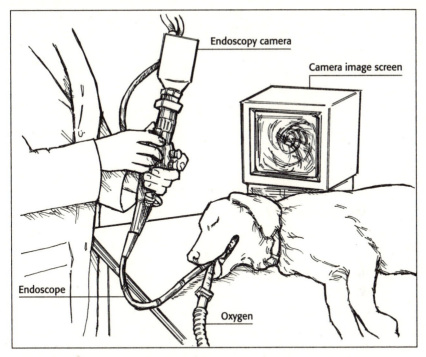

Endoscopy camera

Camera image screen

Endoscope

Oxygen

A dog undergoing upper gastrointestinal endoscopy under general anesthesia. The endoscope is passed through the mouth down the esophagus, and from there into the stomach and small intestine. A tube has been placed in the trachea to administer oxygen and anesthetic gas.

nician and I can place a stomach tube with the endoscope in just a few moments, and our clients find using the tube much easier than forcing food into their pets.

Endoscopy can also be used to diagnose and treat animals who have a stricture, or narrowing, in the esophagus, usually as a result of scar formation due to previous esophageal inflammation or trauma. For example, imagine a dog who swallows a bone that then gets stuck in his esophagus. Due to pressure and injury from the bone, the esophagus can become badly ulcerated. When the ulcer heals, a scar may form, closing off the passage. Using endoscopy, the passage can be opened with specialized balloons that dilate the narrowed area.

Who performs it?

Internal medicine specialists have advanced training and knowledge not only in the performance of endoscopy but also in the interpretation

The Story of Jasmine

Jasmine came to see me because she was not eating and her owner was very worried. When I examined her, I could see that she was jaundiced (her gums and eyes were yellow). Blood tests and an ultrasound exam indicated that Jasmine was likely suffering from hepatic lipidosis, or fatty liver, a condition seen in cats who are stressed or sick and stop eating. It turned out that Jasmine's owner had a nervous guest who was frightened at the thought of a cat walking around while she slept; she would not let Jasmine rest during the day, hoping the cat would sleep all night! She had caused Jasmine so much stress that she became very ill. Fatty liver can be fatal if the cat does not get lots of nutrition right away.

To confirm the diagnosis, we performed a liver biopsy with a needle through the skin using ultrasound guidance. That way, Jasmine avoided surgery, which would have been dangerous in her weakened state. At the same time, we placed a stomach tube in her side using the endoscope. Her owner was happy to see that this did not require surgery, either. Jasmine's owner fed her lots of high-calorie food through the stomach tube at home until the cat's liver healed and she felt like eating again. Needless to say, the guest was not invited back!

and treatment of the results (since gastroenterology is part of internal medicine).

Endoscopy equipment can be purchased easily, and it is important to ensure that the doctor performing endoscopy on your pet is fully qualified. For example, it takes education and experience to develop the ability to pass the endoscope from the stomach into the intestine, especially in small animals. Untrained individuals may examine only the stomach and miss key diagnostic information. It also takes skill to get useful biopsy samples, which requires knowledge of proper biopsy technique and the ability to maneuver the endoscope in very tight spaces. Unfortunately, inadequate biopsies can lead to misdiagnoses.

What are the risks?

Upper GI endoscopy and colonoscopy require general anesthesia in animals. The procedure itself also carries certain risks, depending on the specific situation, and you should discuss this with your doctor. The GI

The Story of Noah

Noah was a cat I treated for an esophageal stricture. When Noah began regurgitating everything he ate, his owner took him to the veterinarian, who referred Noah to me for endoscopic examination of his upper GI tract.

When we looked in his esophagus with the endoscope, we saw that halfway down the passage was almost completely closed. There was a tiny opening not much bigger than a pinhole. Noah's owner agreed that we should use the special dilating balloons to try to help him.

When we use balloons to dilate a strictured area, we do it slowly over several days or weeks, using slightly bigger balloons each time. If we tried to dilate the area to the normal diameter all at once, we might tear the esophagus. In Noah's case, however, the opening was smaller than even our tiniest balloon. What to do? We used the endoscopic biopsy instrument, which is very slender, to push carefully through the hole and make it just big enough to pass the first balloon. Little by little over the next few weeks (while Noah ate only a liquid diet), we carefully dilated Noah's esophagus back to normal.

Why did this happen to him? We never knew. Perhaps he ate something rough or caustic that scarred his esophagus, or a bone became stuck and then passed through. Noah wouldn't tell.

tract can tear during the procedure, requiring surgery. For most animals, this risk is very low.

Respiratory Tract (Bronchoscopy)

Bronchoscopy is endoscopy of the respiratory tract, allowing examination from the larynx (voice box) and trachea (windpipe) to the bronchial tubes in the lungs. The bronchoscope enters through the patient's mouth and then passes through the larynx and down into the lungs.

When would a pet need this?

Bronchoscopy can be used to evaluate the respiratory tract in animals who have symptoms such as coughing, wheezing, or abnormal breathing, or when an abnormality is seen on a radiograph. It can be used to diagnose a variety of conditions, including infections, inflammation, tumors, and abnormal anatomy. It can also be used to locate and remove objects that are caught in an airway.

Who performs it?

Internal medicine specialists, who have advanced knowledge of diseases of the respiratory system.

What are the risks?

Bronchoscopy requires general anesthesia. Risks from the procedure itself include increased coughing, airway irritation, or difficulty breathing after the procedure. There is also a low risk of infection.

Nose (Rhinoscopy)

Rhinoscopy is endoscopy of the inside of an animal's nose and the surrounding tissues. The rhinoscope enters through the animal's nostrils, and both nasal passages are examined, as well as the palate and sometimes the sinuses.

When would a pet need this?

Rhinoscopy is used to examine the nasal passages in animals who have symptoms such as sneezing or snorting, nasal discharge, nosebleeds, noisy or blocked breathing, and swelling of the nose or face. It is used to diagnose infections, inflammation, parasites, and tumors within the nasal cavity, as well as anatomical abnormalities that are causing problems for the animal. It can also be used to locate and remove objects, such as a piece of grass, that have lodged in the nose.

Rhinoscopy may also be used in the treatment of animals who have fungal infections of the nose or sinuses. In some forms of treatment, rhinoscopy is used to clean out the infection and then place medication in the affected areas.

Who performs it?

Internal medicine specialists usually perform rhinoscopy. Some surgeons do as well, particularly those who have a special interest in nasal surgery. Both types of specialists diagnose and treat diseases of the nose and sinuses, sometimes as a team.

What are the risks?

Rhinoscopy requires general anesthesia. There may be some bleeding after the procedure, and patients are often kept overnight so they will rest and remain quiet.

Urogenital Tract (Cystoscopy, Urethroscopy, Vaginoscopy)

Cystoscopy and urethroscopy are endoscopic examinations of the bladder and urethra. The urethra is the passage that urine travels through from the bladder to outside the body. Depending on the equipment available, these procedures can be performed on most dogs and cats (male cats are more challenging due to the small size of their urethra). Vaginoscopy is examination of the vagina and cervix in females.

When would a pet need this?

Endoscopy is a noninvasive way to examine the urinary and reproductive tracts in animals who have a variety of conditions and symptoms, including blood in the urine or straining to urinate, urinary incontinence, frequent urinary tract infections, and unexplained bleeding. This type of procedure is also often used when an animal is suspected of having a congenital abnormality such as ectopic ureters. Ureters are the tiny tubes that carry urine from the kidneys to the bladder. Some animals are born with ureters that do not enter the bladder at the proper location, resulting in incontinence and other problems. Although other methods can be used to diagnose ectopic ureters, endoscopy is currently the best method for doing so with the most accuracy.

Endoscopy can be used to obtain biopsies of a tumor that has been found in the bladder, urethra, or vaginal area, or to look for suspected tumors that are not seen by other methods. For animals with urinary incontinence, there are endoscopic procedures that can be performed to treat the incontinence, such as collagen injections. Animals with urinary tract symptoms will usually have other diagnostics that do not require anesthesia, such as ultrasound scanning, before endoscopy is considered.

Who performs it?

Internal medicine specialists often perform these procedures. Some surgeons do as well, particularly those with a special interest in urinary tract surgery.

The conditions diagnosed and treated using these procedures often lie in an area of overlap between medicine and surgery. For example, a puppy with urinary incontinence may be referred to an internist and diagnosed with ectopic ureters, which require surgery to repair.

What are the risks?

These procedures require general anesthesia. There is risk of tearing the urinary tract, which sometimes requires surgery to repair. There is also risk of infection from the procedure, and antibiotics are often given to help prevent this from occurring. There may be blood in the urine for several hours or days after the procedure.

Thorax (Thoracoscopy)

Thoracoscopy is endoscopy inside the chest cavity. This procedure can be used for the diagnosis and treatment of diseases inside the chest, and also allows minimally invasive surgery to be performed. Several small incisions are made to allow the endoscope and other instruments to be passed into the chest.

When would a pet need this?

Examples include pets with fluid in the chest cavity or around the heart, tumors of the lung or elsewhere in the chest, enlarged lymph nodes in the chest, and lungs that leak air. Some types of congenital heart disease can be repaired using thoracoscopy. It can also be used to obtain biopsies of abnormalities such as tumors and, in some cases, to remove the abnormalities.

Who performs it?

Internal medicine specialists often perform thoracoscopy. Some surgeons do as well, particularly those with a special interest in thoracic surgery.

What are the risks?

The risks of thoracoscopy include trauma to the lungs or elsewhere in the chest and internal bleeding. This procedure requires general anesthesia, with the risks varying depending on the patient and situation. Special types of anesthesia and assisted breathing may be required. You should discuss your pet's particular risks with the doctor performing the procedure.

Abdominal Cavity (Laparoscopy)

Laparoscopy is endoscopy of the abdominal cavity. This procedure allows the abdominal cavity and the organs within to be examined, and minimally invasive surgery to be performed. In many cases, laparoscopy can replace traditional surgery for the evaluation and biopsy of abdominal organs, as well as other surgical procedures. Laparoscopy causes the animal less discomfort and requires a shorter recovery time. In some situations, it is also safer. For example, some animals have conditions that reduce their ability to heal, and laparoscopy requires less healing than traditional surgery. Since laparoscopy involves much smaller incisions, it may also be safer for animals who might bleed excessively due to certain medical conditions.

Laparoscopy requires two or more small incisions to be made to allow the scope and other instruments to enter the abdomen.

When would a pet need this?

Laparoscopy can be used to examine and biopsy the organs. For example, an animal who has abnormal liver enzymes on a blood test could have a liver biopsy performed this way. Laparoscopy can be used for elective surgeries such as ovariohysterectomy (spay), or castration of males in whom one or both testicles have failed to descend and remain in the abdomen.

It is also used for other surgeries, such as removal of the gallbladder, removal of a diseased adrenal gland, removal of bladder stones, or to tack down the stomach (this is sometimes desired in dogs whose stomachs have bloated and twisted, a condition called gastric dilatation and volvulus).

One very worthwhile use of laparoscopy is in animals who are suspected of having metastatic cancer in the abdomen. Traditional surgery often results in a heartbreaking dilemma: If metastatic cancer is indeed found during the operation, the owner may decide to have the pet euthanized while still under anesthesia rather than wake up in discomfort and spend her last days or weeks recovering. With laparoscopy, it is possible to definitively diagnose metastatic cancer without invasive surgery, and allow the pet to spend her remaining time at home with her family.

Who performs it?

Surgeons and internal medicine specialists both perform laparoscopy. Which specialist is used often depends on the procedure that's needed. For example, internists treat disease of the liver and may use laparoscopy to obtain a biopsy. When laparoscopy is used to perform operations (gallbladder removal, for example), this is often done by surgeons. Some general veterinarians also use laparoscopy for certain surgeries, including routine spays.

What are the risks?

Laparoscopy requires sedation or general anesthesia. There are some risks associated with inflating the abdomen, including difficulty with breathing or poor blood flow, air embolism, air under the skin or in abdominal tissues, rupture of the abdomen or diaphragm, and collapsed lungs. Other risks include bleeding and organ trauma. Although this list sounds frightening, when a skilled doctor performs the procedure, the risks are low.

Joints (Arthroscopy)

Arthroscopy is endoscopic examination and treatment of the joints. Many of us are familiar with arthroscopy from personal experience or from hearing about the procedure in human athletes. This procedure has revolutionized the practice of orthopedics, allowing detailed examination of the joints as well as minimally invasive surgery with greatly reduced discomfort and recovery time.

Arthroscopy requires several small incisions to be made to allow the scope and other instruments to enter the joint.

When would a pet need this?

A pet displaying symptoms of joint disease, such as limping, stiffness, difficulty climbing stairs or other obstacles, joint swelling or pain, or joint abnormalities seen on radiographs, may be a candidate for arthroscopy. Arthroscopy is used to diagnose a wide variety of joint conditions and also to surgically treat some of these conditions, particularly developmental joint diseases (those occurring in growing animals).

Who performs it?

Surgeons have training in the techniques used in the procedure, as well as advanced knowledge of the orthopedic diseases that are diagnosed and treated in this way.

What are the risks?

Arthroscopy requires general anesthesia. Nonlife-threatening risks include damage to the cartilage or other joint structures, fluid accumulation around the joint secondary to fluid used during the procedure, and the potential for infection.

Intracranial (Neuroendoscopy)

Neuroendoscopy is endoscopy of the brain. This is a relatively new procedure in veterinary medicine that will continue to develop over time. It has been used with success in a small number of veterinary patients.

When would a pet need this?

Neuroendoscopy has been used to assist in the removal or biopsy of brain tumors and other abnormalities. It has also been used to place drainage tubes in animals with hydrocephalus, a congenital condition of increased fluid in the brain that is particularly common in certain small purebred dogs.

Who performs it?

Neurologists.

What are the risks?

It may be too soon to answer this question, but pets who have undergone neuroendoscopy so far have not experienced significant complications.

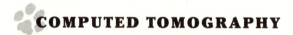COMPUTED TOMOGRAPHY

Computed tomography, also called CT or CAT scan, uses X-ray images taken from many different angles around the patient, which are then processed on a computer to show cross-sectional slices of the body.

Think of a CT scan this way: Imagine dividing a loaf of bread into many thin slices to see what kinds of fruits and nuts it contains. The loaf of bread is the body, and the raisins and walnuts are the organs inside. CT creates images of successive slices of the body area being examined so that abnormalities can be better visualized.

When would a pet need this?

CT has many uses in veterinary medicine. Some of the more common ones include detection of abnormalities of the brain, such as tumors (although MRI is considered superior for this purpose, it is not available for pets in all areas); evaluation of the nasal cavity and sinuses; and detection of very small abnormalities that would not be visible on a regular X-ray. A common example is metastatic cancer in the lungs; even if it is too small to be seen on an X-ray, it may still be picked up by CT.

CT is also used to determine whether a tumor is operable, and to help plan for surgery. CT is much more accurate for these purposes than a regular X-ray. On radiographs, a tumor can only be seen from a few angles and will often be obscured by the surrounding tissues. In contrast, the CT scan will show slices all the way through the tumor and beyond. By looking at a CT scan of the area, the surgeon knows exactly where the tumor begins and ends. For the same reason, CT scans are used by radiation therapists in precisely targeting the location to be treated.

Who performs it?

- Radiologists receive the most education regarding the technology of CT scans, and the most training at interpreting the results.

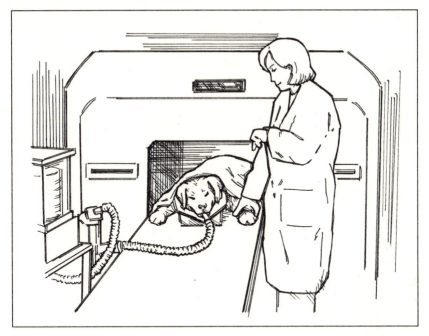

A dog having a CT scan performed. A tracheal tube is in place to administer oxygen and gas anesthetic.

- Neurologists often use CT scans to examine the brain.

- Surgeons use CT to plan operations and diagnose certain conditions.

- Internists use CT to examine various body parts, particularly the nose and sinuses.

- Oncologists use CT to determine the extent of tumors and look for metastatic cancer.

- Radiation oncologists use CT to plan radiation therapy.

What are the risks?

Similar to X-rays, CT scans expose the patient to a small amount of radiation. Although CT is painless, veterinary patients usually require general anesthesia because they must lie perfectly still (and we have yet to find a way to convince animals to do this). Some CT scans involve the use of contrast agents, substances injected into the bloodstream to enhance the images. A low percentage of patients can have adverse reactions to contrast agents.

MAGNETIC RESONANCE IMAGING (MRI)

Remember atoms and protons from science class? Atoms are the smallest possible amount of an element, and protons are one of the subatomic particles that make up atoms. Hydrogen is the simplest atom, with only one proton. MRI uses a strong magnetic field and pulsed radio frequency waves that cause hydrogen protons in the body to wobble and then relax. As this happens, the protons emit signals, which are then processed by a computer to form images. Unlike radiographs and computed tomography (CT), MRI does not use radiation.

MRI is an excellent way to image the soft tissues of the body, and is superior to CT for the evaluation of the brain and spinal cord. However, it's not always available for veterinary patients.

TIP Many veterinary specialists now use mobile MRI. Because MRI equipment is very expensive and requires specialized facilities, its availability for pets is limited. To make this technology more available to veterinary patients, mobile MRI vehicles travel to various locations where specialists practice. Therefore, your pet's neurologist may tell you she performs MRI on certain days of the week, when the mobile unit is scheduled to be present.

When would a pet need this?

MRI is used most commonly in animals to diagnose diseases of the brain and spinal cord, such as tumors, strokes, and herniated (slipped) spinal disks. It is also used to diagnose other neurological issues, such as diseases of the nerves, and to diagnose and evaluate tumors in various parts of the body. The use of MRI for other purposes in veterinary medicine, such as cardiac and gastrointestinal MRI, is being developed.

Who performs it?

- Neurologists most often employ MRI, since it is commonly used to diagnose problems in the brain and spinal cord.

- Radiologists are trained in the interpretation of MRI and are often asked to evaluate an MRI for other specialists.

Depending on the situation, MRI may be used by a variety of specialists, such as oncologists, radiation oncologists, surgeons, criticalists, internal medicine specialists, and cardiologists.

What are the risks?

When used for pets, MRI requires general anesthesia. MRI may involve the use of contrast agents, substances injected into the bloodstream

The Story of Ben

A colleague who is a talented veterinary neurologist recently shared with me the story of her patient Ben. Ben was a three-year-old Lab mix weighing in at over one hundred pounds. Let's face it: Ben was not a slim fellow. One day when chasing a ball in the backyard, he let out a yelp and fell down. His owners ran to help him up, but Ben had suddenly become paralyzed in his rear end and could not use his hind legs.

Ben's owners rushed him to the emergency hospital in their area. The veterinarian at this facility, realizing that time could be of the essence if Ben had an injury to his spinal cord, referred him to the neurologist immediately. The neurologist evaluated Ben and determined that he had indeed suffered severe trauma to his spinal cord. Based on the history, the most likely scenario was that one of the disks in Ben's back had suddenly herniated, damaging his spinal cord and causing paralysis.

Most of the time, rapid herniation of a spinal disk will cause dangerous compression of the spinal cord. If the pressure is not relieved immediately through emergency surgery, permanent paralysis can occur. Ben needed an MRI to evaluate his spinal cord right away. The MRI showed something very interesting: Although one of the disks in his back had indeed herniated and caused the problem, it had virtually exploded; the spinal cord was swollen from the blow it had suffered, but there was no compression of the cord since the disk material was so scattered.

Surgery would not help in Ben's case. Instead, his situation called for an intensive physical therapy regimen, which was begun immediately. Within two days, he was able to move his legs, and within ten days he could walk again.

to enhance the images. A low percentage of patients can have adverse reactions to contrast agents. No radiation is used for MRI.

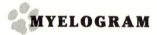

MYELOGRAM

A myelogram is a special type of X-ray of the spinal cord. Because the spinal cord cannot be seen on regular X-rays, a dye is injected into the fluid-filled space surrounding the spinal cord. The dye highlights spinal abnormalities, such as herniated (slipped) disks and tumors.

Myelograms, which always involve general anesthesia, are performed via a spinal tap in either of two locations: the lower back (lumbar) or the neck (cervical). Sometimes dye is injected in both locations.

In human medicine, MRI has largely replaced myelograms. In veterinary medicine, MRI is not always available or affordable, although it is preferred if feasible.

When would a pet need this?

This procedure is performed in pets who are experiencing pain or neurological problems due to disease in the spine. Common examples are slipped disks, tumors, and spinal trauma. Myelograms are used to diagnose the type of spinal condition, the specific location on the spine, and whether or not it is operable. Time is of the essence when treating spinal problems, or permanent paralysis can result.

Who performs it?

- Neurologists.

- Surgeons who perform neurosurgery.

- Radiologists may help interpret the results.

What are the risks?

Myelograms require general anesthesia. Risks include headache, seizures, slowed heart rate, temporary or permanent suspension of breathing, worsening of neurological symptoms, infections, and damage from the needle used for the dye injection. There are fewer complications with lumbar puncture than cervical.

NUCLEAR SCINTIGRAPHY

Nuclear medicine is a branch of medicine that uses radioactive substances to diagnose and treat disease. Within this branch, scintigraphy is a diagnostic tool in which images are created based on the detection of energy from a radioactive substance given to the patient. The substance may be given by injection or other ways, including by mouth or enema. Based on the type used and how it is given, the substance will travel to a specific organ. The radiation emitted by the substance is detected by a special machine, most commonly a type called a gamma camera.

When would a pet need this?

Scintigraphy helps determine the diagnosis and prognosis of a variety of conditions. The most common uses of scintigraphy in veterinary medicine are for thyroid problems, bone cancer, liver shunts, and kidney disease.

Scintigraphy of the thyroid is most frequently used to diagnose an overactive thyroid gland in cats, but can also be used to investigate thyroid cancer and other thyroid conditions.

For pets with bone cancer, scintigraphy is used to detect metastasis (spread) of the cancer. Among other advantages, scintigraphy can detect bony changes before they would be visible on a radiograph.

Liver shunts are abnormal blood vessels that allow the blood to bypass the liver, resulting in toxin buildup that can cause neurological and other symptoms. Animals are sometimes born with these abnormal blood vessels, and scintigraphy may be recommended to help diagnose this problem.

It is also used to assess the function of each kidney—for example, in animals suspected of having early kidney failure that cannot be confirmed by other methods. Or if one kidney may need to be surgically removed (such as a kidney with stones or a tumor), it's helpful to know how well the other kidney is working. Blood tests can't provide this information, since they assess total kidney function rather than the contribution of the individual kidneys.

Scintigraphy can also be used to detect other problems such as adrenal tumors, or to evaluate organ function, including stomach movement, lung function, or possible blockage of the gallbladder. It is not widely available, and is most often found at some veterinary schools and referral centers.

Who performs it?

Radiologists.

What are the risks?

Scintigraphy exposes the patient to a very small amount of radiation, similar to a regular X-ray. Many types of scintigraphy do not require sedation or anesthesia, though some may. Since there are numerous varieties of scintigraphy, specific risks must be discussed with the doctor performing the procedure.

CARDIAC CATHETERIZATION AND ANGIOGRAPHY

Cardiac catheterization and angiography are used to diagnose and treat diseases of the heart and blood vessels. These procedures were more often needed before cardiac ultrasound was developed and refined, but they are still used for certain purposes.

Cardiac catheterization involves inserting a slender plastic catheter into an accessible blood vessel and then advancing it into the heart or a selected blood vessel. Depending on the situation, a dye called a contrast agent may be injected. Angiography involves the use of contrast agents to outline blood vessels. You may be familiar with these procedures in humans for the diagnosis and treatment of atherosclerosis (hardening of the arteries).

When would a pet need this?

One of the most common uses of these procedures is the diagnosis and treatment of some congenital heart defects. For example, a catheterization procedure called balloon valvuloplasty is used to treat a type of heart defect called pulmonic stenosis, where there is partial obstruction of blood flow from the heart into the lungs. In balloon valvuloplasty, a special catheter with a balloon-type tip is used to dilate the narrowed area.

The procedures are also used to measure blood pressure or blood oxygen in specific locations, to evaluate leaky valves or narrowed areas in the heart and blood vessels, and to diagnose and locate blood clots. A similar procedure is used to insert a pacemaker into the heart by threading it through a blood vessel. Pacemakers are used to regulate the heart rate.

Who performs it?

Generally, cardiologists, although radiologists may also be involved in performing the procedure and interpreting results.

What are the risks?

These procedures usually require sedation or anesthesia. If a contrast agent is used, there is a low risk of an adverse reaction. Depending on the procedure and the patient's condition, there may be a risk of the patient developing an abnormal heart rhythm. Other risks include blood loss, blood clots, and damage to the heart or a blood vessel.

As you can see, many types of advanced procedures are available to veterinary patients. The list above is not exhaustive, but should give you an idea of some of the specialized diagnostics that are possible for your pet. As technologies are developed for humans, they are often adapted for use in veterinary medicine (though some are actually used first in animal patients). Continual progress is being made in this area, so the procedures we have discussed will continue to be refined and ever-newer technologies developed.

It's good for concerned pet owners like you to know about these tools. If your pet ever has a health problem, you will know what options are available. As an informed pet owner, you can partner with your veterinarian to find the most skilled doctors and the most cutting-edge technology veterinary medicine has to offer.

This chart illustrates some of the procedures most commonly recommended in pets with various symptoms.

Guide to Diagnostic Procedures by Symptom

Procedures	Appetite decrease	Blood on stool	Breathing abnormality or difficulty	Coughing	Defecation abnormality or difficulty	Diarrhea	Drinking more water	Heart murmur, arrhythmia, or failure	Limping	Nasal discharge or bleeding	Neurological symptoms or behavior changes	Paralysis	Seizures	Sneezing	Urinary abnormality, incontinence, or bleeding	Vomiting	Weight loss
Abdominal ultrasound	•	•			•	•	•								•	•	•
Cardiac ultrasound			•	•				•									
Upper GI endoscopy	•					•										•	•
Colonoscopy		•			•	•											
Bronchoscopy			•	•													
Rhinoscopy			•							•				•			
Cystoscopy															•		
Thoracoscopy			•	•													
Laparoscopy	•					•	•									•	•
Arthroscopy									•								
CT										•	•	•	•	•			
MRI										•		•	•	•			
Myelogram										•		•	•				

SPECIAL PROCEDURES: WORKSHEET

If your pet has been scheduled for a special procedure, you should review the following questions ahead of time, then discuss any concerns with your veterinarian or the specialist(s) performing the procedure.

1. Do I understand what the procedure is?
2. Do I understand why my pet is having the procedure?
3. Does the person performing this procedure have the proper qualifications?
   - Is this person a board-certified specialist in the area?
   - Has this person received formal training in the procedure, such as during a residency program?
   - Is this person experienced with the procedure?

   If the answer to any of these questions is no, is there a veterinarian in my area who is better qualified to perform the procedure?

4. Do I understand all the risks of the procedure?
5. Do I understand all the costs involved in the procedure?
6. Have I been given a written estimate?
7. How much could it cost if something goes wrong during the procedure?

CHAPTER 6

It's Only Natural:

Exploring Alternative Medicine

To many of us, it seems as though our world is becoming progressively less natural in every way. Our food is artificially flavored as often as not. It is irradiated, dyed, frozen, packaged, and preserved. We are woken not by the rising of the sun but by the buzzing of alarms. We spend our days peering at computer screens, communicating with our friends and colleagues via electronic mail, and traveling back and forth encased in air-conditioned pollution-spewing vehicles. Everything around us seems to be made of or covered by plastic. We feel some mixture of concern, guilt, and fatalism about these developments, and although it all seems very worrisome, it is virtually impossible to extricate ourselves from these realities of our current existence without becoming forest-dwelling hermits.

It is little wonder that we feel a desire to get back to nature. This may mean seeking out organically grown foods, spending time in rural settings, or turning to health care modalities that seem to promise more natural-sounding solutions to whatever may ail us or our pets. It is tempting to make medical decisions based on positive or negative symbolism—plants versus chemicals, herbs versus drugs, natural versus synthetic—yet of course it is important that we also look deeper and base our choices on objective reality rather than simply upon appealing icons. This is especially true given that we are constantly pressured by marketing strategies centered on claims that a product or service is more natural.

Many concerned pet owners have questions on this topic as it relates to their pets' health. They want to know: Are herbs and other alternative medical approaches safer than drugs and conventional medicine? Are they as effective? And are they truly more natural for us and for our pets? Are there actually clear demarcations among plants, herbs, and drugs? We will be exploring these types of questions in this chapter. It will also be helpful for us to clearly define and understand various alternative medical approaches. Terms such as *holistic, homeopathic,* and *herbal* are often used interchangeably, although they are not in fact the same things at all.

In this chapter, I'll start out by examining the term *natural* and attempting to understand exactly what we mean when we use it. For concerned pet owners, it is essential to remain informed about the choices that are available regarding our pets' health. We all have a common goal: to make decisions that will benefit our pets and prevent harm to them. Therefore the decisions we make must be based on education and understanding so that we do not inadvertently put our pets at risk in our very quest to keep them safe and well.

What is natural, *and is it better?*

The word *natural* has become so ubiquitous that it has begun to lose any clear meaning. It seems like every product out there claims to be natural, and therefore better. Because I get so many questions from my veterinary clients that in some way involve this term, I have had to think long and hard about what it truly means for something to be natural, and whether those products and services marketed as being more natural are generally better for our pets. I have come to realize that there aren't simple answers to these questions; the situation varies depending on the specific circumstance or product being assessed. Each must be evaluated individually.

When I sat down to really mull over the question of whether things we might think of as being more natural are always better, I started by thinking about our own human lives. When I try to picture the "natural" life of a human being, the cavemen generally come to mind. They lived completely natural lives, without heat, hot water, cooked food, or fluoride toothpaste, and had an average life span of less than twenty years (compared with our expected life span of almost eighty years). During their short lives, they likely spent a good part of their time too cold, too hot, hungry, sick, or with a terrible toothache! So in the purest sense, few of us would choose to go back to a natural human life. How many of us would elect to give up toothpaste, refrigeration, electricity, or antibiotics? Or how about central heating, telephones, showers, or toilets?

Since my life is devoted to caring for pets, I have also considered what a natural life for them might entail. According to studies, unowned cats live an average of about one and a half years outdoors—not exactly what we would choose for our own feline companions. Our dogs' relatives, the gray wolves, live an average of five or six years in the wild. Our expectations regarding our pet canines generally involve a life span at least double that. When I think about these statistics, I have to recognize that natural might not always be better, at least for the individual. In fact, I wouldn't actually want my dog or cat to live a natural life, because it would involve a lot more fear, hunger, injury, and illness, and a much shorter life span than my beloved pets experience!

The truth is that a lot of the things we might be tempted to label as unnatural, including medical advances such as anesthesia and antibiotics, allow us and our pets to live a lot longer and a heck of a lot more comfortably. We're living longer all the time, and conquering more diseases every year. To say that we want our pets to truly live naturally would mean denying them all the advances that we humans have come to rely on and even take for granted. I don't think any of us would want that. What we really want is for our pets to be healthy and safe, and we are all seeking the best ways to accomplish that goal.

Regarding different ways of practicing medicine, it's not easily feasible to define what is natural. If herbs are natural, are they still so when grown using pesticides, processed on factory machinery, compressed into tablets, packaged in plastic containers, then stored for months or years? If plants are natural, what about drugs extracted from plants, or medications based on substances originally found in plants but produced more safely and economically when synthesized? We also cannot assume that something that occurs in nature is always beneficial. Many plants and minerals are poisonous, or are toxic to one particular species. Lilies cause kidney failure in cats, and grapes can do the same in dogs. These plants are natural, but they are harmful to our pets.

After much consideration, I've decided that it isn't really useful, and may be impossible, to define what is now natural and apply it to our pets, or to decide if everything marketed as natural is actually better. Instead, I try to rationally evaluate what treatment plan will be healthiest and best for each individual animal, based on objective evidence. I don't choose my patients' medication by how appealing the label is, but by our understanding of its safety and effectiveness.

What can we learn from the way our pets' ancestors lived or the way wild animals live in nature?

For me, as a veterinarian whose goal is to keep my patients as healthy and happy as possible, the best use of our knowledge about what was natural for our pets' ancestors is as an educational tool that we can learn from and build upon. In other words, nature is a great starting point to understand how our pets evolved, which can teach us much about how to best feed and care for them. So although I wouldn't want my pets or patients to live the short, perilous life of a wild animal, I do use my knowledge about their ancestors' lives to help me take better care of them.

For instance, we can learn much about the best ways to feed animals from the diet of their ancestors. This matters because we know that our pets' modern physiology is based on the environment their ancestors inhabited. Cats, for example, evolved based on a very specific environment and food source, and this cannot be ignored when designing diets for modern cats. It's not that their ancestors' diet was inherently good; it's that the physiology of cats adapted to fit the diet that was then available, and ignoring this today can be dangerous.

The predecessors of our domestic cats dwelled in the desert. They lived entirely on prey, and got all of their fluids from their prey as well. Because of this, cats are able to conserve water by making their urine extremely concentrated, and they don't get as thirsty as some other species when they are dehydrated. These adaptations were very useful in the desert, but now predispose cats to certain health problems such as forming urinary crystals due to their highly concentrated urine and tolerance of dehydration. We can help combat this by feeding them in ways that supply more fluid. Since cats' ancestors obtained their liquid from their food, our cats' bodies don't understand that on a dry diet they need to drink much more water to make up for the deficit. Due to their desert-based physiology, cats on dry diets simply take in less fluid, which can be risky.

Cats' naturally completely carnivorous diet led to a metabolism based on animal protein; dietary carbohydrates are not natural for them, and can lead to issues such as diabetes and obesity. Due to their status as pure carnivores (unlike dogs whose physiology is more nutritionally flexible), cats cannot utilize nutrients from plants the way dogs and humans can. They are unable, for example, to convert plant beta-carotene to vitamin A as we do. Instead, cats must ingest vitamin A directly from animal tissue.

This brings up another important point: Something that is healthy or natural for us is not necessarily the best thing for our pets. Because we all know that fruits and vegetables are very good for human beings, we could make the mistake of thinking they are equally good for our feline friends. In fact, cats' metabolisms have no need for plant matter, and they cannot utilize vegetable nutrients the way we do. If cats were fed the healthiest diet for a human being, they would be very unhealthy indeed, while if we ate the natural diet of a cat, we would risk severely high cholesterol, clogged arteries, and heart attacks!

Our pets do pay the price when we ignore their physiologic evolution. This was seen starkly when thousands of cats developed heart failure due to a deficiency in cat food of taurine, an amino acid cats rely on that is naturally found only in animal tissue. Now taurine is routinely added to cat food, but we still gamble with our cats' health by feeding them high-carbohydrate dry diets based in large part on grain meal. Luckily dogs are more forgiving: Like us, they are omnivorous, and they can adjust to different types of food sources.

The goal is not to re-create nature, but to learn from it . . .

I don't think we would do our pets any favors by trying to turn back the clock and have them lead the lives their ancestors did—brief ones full of deprivation, danger, and disease. At the same time, there is much to be learned by what occurs in nature. We can learn what may be good and also what is clearly bad for our pets. In nature, dogs and cats die of infectious disease; thus we vaccinate our pets. In nature, eating raw animal tissue leads to parasitic infestation, so we cook our pets' food to protect them from parasites and harmful bacteria. In nature, ticks spread disease, so we have developed products to protect our pets from tick bites and tick-borne disease. In nature, dogs and cats are infected with heartworms, so we test our pets and give them a monthly preventive. It is natural for wild animals to be parasite-ridden and to quickly succumb to age or any disease that afflicts them, but we shield our pets from natural hazards by protecting them from parasites and infections, by caring for them in their old age, and by treating diseases that affect them.

Is alternative medicine more natural or safer than conventional medicine?

The best approach to this question is for you to become well educated about various types of alternative medical approaches, and to then decide for yourself. As far as safety is concerned, keep in mind as we explore this topic that there are two kinds of safety: the absence of direct harm (such as injury or toxicity) and the presence of effectiveness. One question that you must always consider is whether by choosing a particular medical approach for your pet, you have forgone another that might have been more beneficial.

For example, if in lieu of an antibiotic, you give your pet who has pneumonia an herbal supplement that promises to fight infection, and the herb causes no side effects but does not effectively treat your pet's pneumonia, was it safe? In one sense, it was: It did not directly injure your pet. However, if the hope of the herb working convinced you to reject the antibiotic, and your pet continues to be ill or even succumbs to the infection, it may not have been safe after all. Proven effectiveness is an essential parameter that must not be forgotten when judging the safety of any health care product.

I believe that when making health care choices for our pets, it is advisable for us to base our choices on education and evidence. In other words, I prefer to approach the practice of medicine rationally, and to be sure that any treatment I recommend for a patient or use on my own pet will be safe and effective, regardless of the source. Because a particular treatment might seem at first glance more natural does not mean that it is useful or even harmless for dogs and cats. At the same time, a medical modality should not be rejected simply because it may be unconventional. I prefer to keep an open mind, investigate the evidence, and decide based on facts what may benefit my patients. I also always keep in mind species differences, and remember that evidence regarding one species cannot be extrapolated to another. What is good for a human may not be good for a dog or a cat, and what is safe in one species may well be highly toxic in another.

*I want to protect my pet's health. What type of evidence is
necessary to prove that a particular treatment is safe or effective?*

To protect your pet, it's important for you to understand how we learn
whether a proposed medical treatment is useful or safe. Most doctors
(human or veterinary) feel it is best to practice what's called evidence-
based medicine. This refers to medical treatments that have been objectively evaluated through carefully performed clinical trials; without this
type of appropriate analysis, it is very easy to draw the wrong conclusions.
If consumers don't understand how appropriate studies are conducted, it
can seem as though a product has indeed been shown to be safe or effective, even when this is not truly the case.

Let's perform our own theoretical study to illustrate how this is cor-
rectly done, and also how tempting it can be to draw inaccurate conclusions. We'll perform an imaginary clinical trial to see if vitamin E is an
effective treatment for dogs who have itchy skin. How will we go about
this?

Control group: We'll need to have two groups of dogs—the itchy dogs
who receive vitamin E, and also what's called a control group. This is a
group of patients who either do not receive the treatment being studied or
receive a different one, so that a comparison can be made. If we simply
gave twenty itchy dogs vitamin E, and they all eventually stopped scratching, we might claim that vitamin E is a great treatment for itchy dogs. But
that wouldn't be right: We must also have another twenty itchy dogs who
do *not* receive vitamin E. If these dogs also stop scratching at some point
(as most dogs eventually do), that might suggest that it wasn't really the vitamin E that helped, but perhaps just the passage of time, the dogs' own
immune systems, or even a change in the weather.

Suppose that it took an average of two weeks for the dogs in the control group to scratch less, but that the dogs who received vitamin E seemed
better to their owners after an average time of only one week. Now we're
getting somewhere; now *maybe* we can say that vitamin E does help itchy
dogs.

Blinding: Why do I say that *maybe* vitamin E helped the dogs? After all,
the dogs on vitamin E stopped scratching a week faster, on average, than
those who didn't get this therapy. Well, the reason that I say *maybe* is
what's called the placebo effect. This refers to the fact that the owners of
the dogs who got vitamin E may have believed or wanted to believe that

the vitamin made their dogs feel better, and their evaluation of their dogs' condition may have been affected by this belief. The placebo effect is very powerful, and can work in various ways. If the pet owners participating in the study knew that we were studying the effectiveness of vitamin E for itchy dogs, this could influence the information they report to us. For example, they might subconsciously want to please us by saying that their dogs seemed less itchy. Their optimism regarding the treatment might cause them to truly believe their dogs were showing improvement. The dogs' behavior may also be affected if they sense their owners' enthusiasm.

To make the study accurate, we must make sure that the dog owners don't know what they are giving—we'll use identical capsules that contain either vitamin E or just sugar, and we won't tell the owners which we have given them. That's called a blinded study, because it's sort of as though all the subjects were wearing blindfolds. Now if the owners report more improvement in those dogs who are truly receiving the vitamin, maybe we can say that vitamin E helps itchy dogs.

Randomization: At this point, you probably want to scream. *Maybe* vitamin E helps itchy dogs? It seems definite now! Well, actually, no. There is another variable we need to control. We need our study to be randomized.

You see, we need to talk about how we decided who would get real vitamin E and who would get sugar capsules. What if all the owners came into a room with their dogs, and our research assistant handed out the capsules to them? And what if the assistant happens to like big dogs, and so she gave the real vitamin E to all the big dogs' owners? What if she did it without even realizing it? And what if big dogs just tend to be less itchy than little dogs? Now our study results won't be accurate.

We need to randomize the study by making sure that the research assistant puts all the owners' names in a hat, then pulls out twenty names for vitamin E and twenty names for sugar capsules without looking. Now we can be sure that it is truly random which dogs get vitamin E and which dogs get sugar capsules. Another way to fix this issue is to perform what's called a double-blind study. In a double-blind study, not only are the dog owners unaware of whether they are getting vitamin E or just sugar capsules, but the research assistant is also unaware of which one she is handing to each person. The capsules might be in containers simply labeled A or B, for example.

You can see from our little experiment that it's fairly easy for it to *look* like a treatment worked whether it truly did or not. Without a control group, blinding, and randomization, study results are easy to misinterpret. But there should be firm and objective evidence that a therapy is both safe and effective before it is used on people's pets. No matter which medical approach a doctor or veterinarian uses, it should be held to these same standards. Unfortunately, there are very few studies in veterinary patients investigating the various types of alternative medicine. This makes it much more difficult to say whether particular alternative treatments are safe or helpful. Hopefully, one day we will have more information.

In discussing alternative approaches to veterinary medicine, I'm going to first address some general questions. Then I'll describe some of the more popular alternative medical modalities, talk about any existing evidence regarding each approach in pets, and attempt to give you some practical guidelines in light of what is currently known about the safety and usefulness of that approach for pets.

What is complementary and alternative medicine?

According to the National Center for Complementary and Alternative Medicine (NCCAM), a division of the National Institutes of Health (NIH), complementary and alternative medicine (CAM) is "a group of diverse medical and health care systems, practices, and products that are not presently considered to be part of conventional medicine. While some scientific evidence exists regarding some CAM therapies, for most there are key questions that are yet to be answered through well-designed scientific studies—questions such as whether these therapies are safe, and whether they work for the diseases or medical conditions for which they are used."

What's the difference between alternative medicine and complementary medicine?

Alternative medicine is used in place of conventional medicine. Complementary medicine, as the name implies, is used along with conventional medicine.

What about holistic medicine?

The word *holistic* is a descriptive term that refers to a focus on the whole rather than the parts. Since any good doctor assesses and treats the entire patient, this term does not refer to any specific branch of medicine. For example, when a thorough veterinarian treats a dog with allergic skin disease, she not only prescribes medication to ease the itching but also attempts to discover what element in the dog's environment or food is stimulating the problem, uses a special diet if indicated, and takes measures to prevent the allergic reaction from recurring in the future. Holism simply means that disease processes must be viewed in context, and this should always be the case.

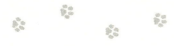

There are many alternative medical approaches offered in veterinary medicine. Three of the most popular are herbal medicine, acupuncture, and homeopathy. Let's explore these individually.

HERBAL MEDICINE

What Are Herbs?

According to the NCCAM, an herb is "a plant or plant part used for its scent, flavor, and/or therapeutic properties." Pet owners may purchase and give herbs to their pets on their own, or veterinarians practicing alternative medicine may recommend or dispense herbal products. Herbs may also be used as one component of certain alternative medical systems, such as traditional Chinese medicine (TCM) or Indian ayurvedic medicine. In TCM, herbs are often combined into formulas containing multiple herbs and other nonherbal substances, such as minerals or animal parts.

Herbs are sometimes assumed to be more natural or safer alternatives to drugs. In actuality, herbs and drugs are closely related; in fact drugs are often purified or synthetic forms of active substances found in plants. More than a hundred current drugs are plant-derived, including the heart medication digoxin, the painkiller and cough suppressant codeine, the anti-gout drug colchicine, the Parkinson's drug L-dopa, the anti-tumor drug Taxol, the bronchial tube dilator theophylline, the chemotherapy drugs vincristine and vinblastine, and good old aspirin.

The Difference Between Herbs and Drugs

Herbs are whole plants or parts of plants that contain variably active substances, with many such substances often being present within one herb. Herbal supplement products may include several herbs and sometimes other substances as well, and may contain dozens or even hundreds of active ingredients (although the label may only list one or a few). Drugs, on the other hand, generally contain one purified active component. Drugs may be based on substances found in plants, with the desired compound either isolated (so that the drug contains only one active ingredient) or synthesized (manufactured from a source other than the original plant the substance was found in).

The story of aspirin is a perfect illustration of the connection between herbs and drugs, and the evolution of one from the other. Traditionally, willow bark was used as a treatment for fevers, aches, and pains. In the 1800s, the active substance in willow bark, salicin, was isolated. From this came salicylic acid, an earlier form of aspirin. Later, it was discovered that a related compound, acetylsalicylic acid, is safer than salicylic acid, with fewer side effects. Acetylsalicylic acid is the active ingredient in modern aspirin. Thus, like many drugs, aspirin is in essence a purified, synthesized herb. Since more than one trillion aspirin tablets have been consumed since its inception, the willow trees are probably grateful that we have learned to make it for ourselves!

Herbs must be treated with respect and caution. As you can see by the list of powerful drugs derived from plants, herbs can be potent and potentially very toxic. To assume that, because an active substance is cloaked with an innocent-sounding plant name, it is therefore harmless is an error. Additionally, herbs may contain many variably active ingredients, and the amounts and strengths of these active ingredients in herbal products are difficult to predict or control. It is important to realize that plants often contain these substances as poisons to deter animals from eating them, and although in controlled, small amounts we use these materials as medications, we must never forget their original, more dangerous purpose in nature.

Some Cautionary Facts About Herbs, Supplements, and Nutraceuticals

Unlike drugs, which are controlled by the FDA and must be approved, herbal products and nutraceuticals are not regulated. They need not undergo a premarket approval process, and there is no guarantee of their safety, effectiveness, or manufacturing process. In other words, you are largely on your own when you purchase or use them. Manufacturers don't have to submit any safety information to the FDA before placing products on the market.

Herbal ingredients and safety will vary based on:

- The part of the plant that is used (roots, stems, leaves, or flowers).

- Climates and growing conditions. When these are inconsistent, different batches—even those manufactured by the same company— can have variable potency and safety.

- Storage conditions and length of storage. These factors are not regulated. Some products don't even have expiration dates on them.

- Proper identification of plants on product labels, which is not always the case.

- The skill of the workers who collect and process the plants. In the most tragic instances, fatal toxicities have occurred when poisonous plants have been harvested in error.

- Type of herb preparation—extract, tablet, capsule, dried herb, and so forth.

- Potential environmental contaminants in the product, including microorganisms (bacteria, fungi, or molds), toxins produced by these microorganisms, heavy metals the plant was exposed to (for example, mercury, cadmium, and lead), pesticides, and insecticides (unless herbs are organically grown).

None of these variables or potential contaminants is regulated. Two different products advertising that they contain the same herb may thus have wildly different levels of safety and/or activity. Another concern is that in multiple instances, herbal supplements have been discovered to be adulterated with prescription medications. This can occur through accidental contamination; in some cases, though, it's done deliberately to make the product appear to be more powerful or effective.

Unlike drug companies, manufacturers of herbs and supplements are not required to report negative events of which they are aware. In other words, an herbal manufacturer could keep silent about any sickness or fatality resulting from use of the product, continuing to market it. Therefore you have no way to know if other people's pets have suffered ill effects from use of a particular herb or supplement. Due to the strict regulation and oversight to which drugs are subject, any negative events in human or animal patients taking a drug must be reported and can lead to withdrawal of the drug from the market.

There is similarly no regulation of the labeling of herbs and supplements. What this means is that there is no oversight as to the accuracy of the labels placed on such products. For example, one study regarding chondroitin sulfate—an ingredient commonly used in products advertised for joint health—found that nine of eleven products claiming to contain chondroitin had inaccurate labels. The percentage error in the listed amount of chondroitin was off by up to 115 percent!

When a company called Consumer Laboratory, which analyzes and validates these types of products, investigated ten different common ingredients, they found that only four were accurately listed on product labels at least 80 percent of the time. (Those four were glucosamine, coenzyme Q, iron, and dimethylsulfone.)

Herbs and supplements can have dangerous interactions with each other and with medications and anesthetic agents, so it is essential to inform your veterinarian of any products you are using in your pet, and to investigate potential interactions before giving a product to your pet. Because herbal products contain inconsistent concentrations of ingredients and diverse parts of the plant, and because people use (on themselves or their pets) varying doses, these interactions are quite difficult to prevent or predict. Here are some examples of adverse interactions.

- St.-John's-wort, found in several pet products, is the most notorious. This herb can decrease the effectiveness of many drugs, such as those used for allergies, autoimmune diseases, heart disease, and bronchial conditions. Because of this effect, the use of St.-John's-wort has caused human transplant patients to reject their transplants: Their anti-rejection drugs lost activity. This same effect resulted in decreased activity of anti-viral drugs in HIV-positive people.

- Valerian, found in several pet products as an herbal sedative, may increase the effects of anesthetics, sedatives, anti-seizure drugs, and painkillers, so it is important to let your veterinarian know if your pet has taken valerian.

- Ginseng can decrease the effects of narcotic painkillers. It should not be used in animals who may be given these drugs for painful procedures or conditions.

- Minerals such as calcium, iron, magnesium, and zinc can reduce the absorption and effectiveness of medications like antibiotics and thyroid supplements. This is also true of herbal formulas and supplements with calcium-rich ingredients, such as oyster shell, mother-of-pearl, and "dragon bone," or other herbal formulas that may be rich in various minerals. Unless you are an expert, this may be hard to ascertain, particularly as many herbal formulas contain multiple, often quite mysterious, ingredients.

- Potassium supplements may increase the risk of potassium toxicity in patients taking certain heart medications and diuretics.

- Echinacea can decrease the activity of chemotherapy or radiation therapy.

- Grapefruit juice, and potentially grapefruit seed extract, can increase levels of certain drugs in the body, leading to potential overdose. Levels of other drugs may be decreased.

- Ginkgo can cause reduction or increase in blood levels and activity of medications. In rodent studies, ginkgo caused blood levels of heart medication to rise, an effect that could lead to drug overdose. On its own, ginkgo has been shown to potentially cause bleeding disorders. Because of this, it should not be used in patients on NSAIDs or blood thinners.

- Garlic supplements have caused bleeding in humans, and garlic has been shown to reduce the function of canine and human platelet cells (the cells that help control bleeding). Garlic should not be used in animals with bleeding tendencies, those on blood thinners, or those having surgery. Garlic may also increase the effects of gas anesthetics, another reason to avoid garlic before surgeries.

- Ginger may also lead to bleeding disorders, particularly in combination with blood thinners.

- Normal doses of vitamin E can cause animals and people on blood thinners to develop bleeding disorders. Overdose of vitamin E by itself can cause decreased blood clotting, leading to hemorrhage.

Because so many herbs can potentially lead to bleeding problems or can interact with anesthetics and painkillers, the American Society of Anesthesiologists advises that all herbs be stopped several weeks before any surgery is performed on a patient. But this is helpful only for patients having planned surgery and will not protect an animal or person who has taken herbal medication and is now undergoing emergency surgery.

As I discussed above, herbs are not subject to the type of regulation and safety mechanisms that govern the manufacture and sale of drugs. Of course this regulation doesn't mean that drugs won't have side effects. It does mean, however, that the concentration of the active ingredient in a drug is consistent; thus doctors generally feel that the results are more effective and predictable and that potential side effects are more restricted and foreseeable. When using a drug, such as aspirin, the doctor or consumer knows the exact ingredients and the milligrams of active substance being taken. When using herbs, no such guarantees exist.

Because drugs are generally given to people and pets under the supervision of a doctor, dosing is consistent and appropriate, and potential interactions can be minimized. Herbs and supplements are for the most part taken by consumers or given to pets without medical oversight. In alternative medical approaches, herbs may be dispensed by a medical professional, and this doctor or veterinarian should carefully monitor the dose, preparation, and potential interactions of any products that are used.

Evidence Regarding Herbs in Dogs and Cats

Unfortunately, very little clinical research has been done on the use of herbs for veterinary patients. Because herbs can be potentially toxic, and because the effects of many substances vary in different species, it is not safe to extrapolate research done in humans to animals. Something that is safe for a person may not be safe for our pets. For example, chocolate is poisonous to dogs, and the commonly used painkiller acetaminophen is extremely toxic to cats. The sweetener xylitol, an ingredient in many products for humans, is highly toxic to dogs. It is just impossible to accurately predict from experience in one species what the effect of a substance will be in another species. It is not even advisable to use data from dogs for cats or vice versa, since the physiology of these two species is so very different. Many substances that are safe for dogs are toxic to cats, and the reverse can be true as well.

A review of human and veterinary medical journals over the past ten years reveals only a few studies of herbs in dogs, and none in cats. A randomized, double-blind, placebo-controlled study described in the journal *Veterinary Dermatology* showed some effectiveness of P07P, a product derived from a traditional Chinese herbal remedy, for dogs with allergic skin disease. A more recent study in the same journal evaluated the related product PYM00217, developed for use in dogs with allergic skin disease and containing three standardized plant extracts, and found it to be effective. Another randomized, double-blind, placebo-controlled study of the formula P54FP, an extract of Indian and Javanese tumeric, showed some possible positive effects on canine arthritis. An article in the *Journal of the American Veterinary Medical Association* reported that supplements containing the herbs guarana and ma huang caused toxicity in dogs, which was fatal in 17 percent of the dogs.

There is no doubt that many herbs are powerful substances, and that some herbs and herbal formulas have been shown to result in particular effects in humans or in experimental animals, most commonly rodents. The problems with using herbs safely and effectively in our pets are:

- So little research has been done using herbs in dogs or cats that it is impossible to accurately determine the safety or effectiveness of most products at this point.

- The herbs and herbal products on the market are so poorly regulated and standardized that even if we knew from scientific studies that a particular herb was potentially effective, it would be very difficult to reliably give an animal a precise dose.

- Because of this poor regulation, it is difficult to ensure that an herbal product does not contain potentially harmful contaminants, such as heavy metals, insecticides, pesticides, or microorganisms.

How can we safely and effectively use herbs in our pets? I am not convinced that we can with our current limited knowledge. Hopefully, our present ignorance will eventually be rectified; improved understanding will require properly designed studies that to date have not been carried out. However, there are some practical guidelines to follow that can help you to keep your pet safe if you are considering the use of herbs:

- Use herbs only under the guidance of a licensed, reputable veterinarian.

- When selecting and evaluating any veterinarian, adhere to the same principles that I discussed in the first chapter to ensure that you have chosen a high-quality practice for your pet. Those standards of care apply no matter what medical approach the particular veterinarian or practice chooses to follow.

- Be sure to tell your veterinarian about all herbs and supplements you have given or are currently giving to your pet. Since there can be potentially dangerous interactions among various herbs or between herbs and drugs, it is essential that you and your veterinarian are in full communication.

- Because many herbs or other ingredients in herbal supplements can affect the activity of medications, leading to decreased effectiveness or even overdose, the use of herbs should be minimized or avoided in pets who are on other medications. This is most important in patients for whom the other medications are essential for health. If herbs and drugs are used in the same patient, they should be taken at separate times, although doing so does not ensure that interaction will not occur.

- The use of herbs should be avoided in pets who will be having surgery, particularly those herbs that are known to predispose to hemorrhage or increase the effects of anesthetics and sedatives.

- For pets with serious health conditions, herbs should not be used as a substitute for proven conventional therapies.

- Pet owners should investigate carefully any herbs they are considering giving to their pet. Because of the lack of regulation in this area, owners should not trust the labels on herbal products for health recommendations for their pets. One helpful avenue is to contact an animal poison control service, such as the ASPCA's Animal Poison Control Center, where veterinary toxicologists are likely to be aware of any known or recent dangers of particular herbal products in pets.

A client of mine recently was considering giving an herbal supplement marketed and labeled as promoting kidney health to her dog, who suffers from chronic renal failure. The supplement contained twenty-two active ingredients. When we contacted the ASPCA's Animal Poison Control Center, the staff strongly advised against using the herbal formula, as many of the ingredients were potentially harmful to the dog's kidneys.

ACUPUNCTURE

Originating in China, acupuncture is a procedure in which thin needles are inserted into the body in order to treat illness or relieve pain. There are various types of acupuncture, such as traditional acupuncture using needles, electroacupuncture using electrical charges, sonoacupuncture using sound waves, and moxibustion using burning herbs. Acupuncture is performed at specific acupuncture points having a high density of nerves and blood vessels. There are different ideas as to how acupuncture works, one prevailing theory being that it causes the release of natural opioids (morphine-like chemicals called endorphins) by the body.

Although there are numerous studies of acupuncture in humans, unfortunately many of these are felt to be of unacceptable quality, since they did not follow the principles of well-designed experiments that I discussed earlier. The effectiveness of acupuncture is controversial in human medicine, with some doctors believing that there is no evidence whatsoever of effectiveness, and others feeling that there is some evidence of the usefulness of acupuncture in certain specific situations, such as for treating arthritis pain and relieving certain types of nausea.

An issue with many studies on the effectiveness of acupuncture is that they did not include a control group of patients who believed they were receiving acupuncture but were not. For example, to study acupuncture's effect on pain, it is important to determine that the acupuncture is not simply acting as a placebo. In fact, it has been suggested that one of the ways acupuncture may work is by the power of suggestion: If people believe strongly enough that it will help them, they actually feel better.

One way to determine if this is occurring is by using a procedure that has been recently developed called sham acupuncture, in which fake needles that appear to penetrate the skin are used for the control group. In this way, researchers can be sure that any apparent effects of acupuncture are not due to a placebo effect. Sham acupuncture can also be used for studies done in pets, to rule out the possibility of the placebo effect on their owners or the researchers who are evaluating the results of the therapy, and also to ensure that simply handling the animals during the procedure is not affecting them in some way (with sham acupuncture, the control group of animals is handled in a similar manner to those who actually receive treatment).

Evidence Regarding Acupuncture in Dogs and Cats

Several studies have been done evaluating the use of acupuncture in pets. In one interesting study published in 2006, a group of veterinarians evaluated the use of electroacupuncture for dogs with elbow arthritis. This study included the use of sham acupuncture for the control group. The authors found no difference in lameness or pain in the dogs who received acupuncture compared with the dogs who did not, so the electroacupuncture was not apparently helpful for the arthritis. However, the dogs' owners were able to guess when their dogs received real acupuncture versus sham acupuncture. The researchers wondered if perhaps the acupuncture made the dogs feel generally better even though it did not help their arthritis, maybe due to the release of endorphins.

An article analyzing the effectiveness of acupuncture in veterinary medicine was published in 2006. The authors reviewed all of the veterinary acupuncture studies that they could find. Some of these studies evaluated the use of acupuncture for artificially induced conditions rather than naturally occurring diseases. For example, the liver or spine of dogs was deliberately damaged, and the effect of acupuncture on this damage was assessed. The authors concluded that many of the studies were of poor quality, and there wasn't yet strong evidence either for or against the use of acupuncture for animals.

Risks of Acupuncture

Acupuncture is generally safe when performed by a well-trained professional. However, it is not completely without risk. Complications that have occurred include local bleeding, nerve damage, and infection if contaminated needles are used. One of the most severe complications that can occur is a punctured lung. If acupuncture is used in lieu of a proven conventional treatment for a life-threatening condition, the risk in this case is of potential ineffectiveness.

HOMEOPATHY

Homeopathy is a very specific alternative medical approach that is based on several quite controversial principles. If you are considering the use of homeopathic remedies for your pet, it is very important that you understand the beliefs upon which homeopathy is based so that you can make informed decisions.

Homeopathy was developed in the 1700s by a German doctor named Samuel Hahnemann, and is based upon the following theories:

The Law of Similars: This concept proposes that a substance causing particular symptoms in healthy individuals can be used to alleviate those same symptoms when caused by illness: "Like cures like." For example, based on this theory, a substance that causes a healthy person or animal to have a runny nose could cure a runny nose caused by disease. Homeopathy derives its name (which is based on two Greek words: *homoios,* meaning "similar," and *pathos,* meaning "suffering") from this principle.

Potentization: This concept holds that when a substance is repeatedly diluted and shaken ("succussed") many times, it becomes more potent. In homeopathy, a remedy that is more dilute, and thus contains less (or often none) of the original substance, is considered to have higher potency.

How Homeopathic Remedies Are Prepared

Homeopathic remedies are generally obtained from plants, animals, and minerals. After the crude substance is extracted from its source, this substance is then diluted repeatedly, being shaken in some manner between each dilution. The number of dilutions is indicated by a combination of Roman and Arabic numerals. For example, a 30X dilution has gone through thirty dilutions of one part in ten. To do this, the substance is diluted to one-tenth of its original strength thirty times, resulting in a solution that is 1,000,000,000,000,000,000,000,000,000,000 times more dilute than the original. A 30C solution has been diluted to a one-hundredth of its strength thirty times, resulting in a solution that is 1,000,000,000,000,000,000,000,000,000,000,000,000,000,000,000,000,000,000,000,000 times more dilute than the original. A 50M solution has been diluted to a one-hundred-thousandth of its strength fifty times (I won't write out the zeros for that one!). The final product of these dilutions is then sprayed on a tiny pill and allowed to dry.

Controversy Regarding Homeopathy

Homeopathic theories and methods have been the subject of much debate and skepticism. Critics have made the following points:

- Homeopathy is based upon the treatment of symptoms rather than the diagnosis and correction of the underlying disease. This has been questioned because similar symptoms are caused by many different conditions, which may require specific therapy. For example, vomiting can be caused by an object lodged in the intestines (which would conventionally be treated by removing the object), a viral infection (which would be treated by hydration and other supportive care), a food allergy (which would be treated by avoiding this food in the future), an ulcer (which would be healed with antacids), and so on.

  The concern has been raised that by treating symptoms rather than attempting to diagnose and treat their cause, homeopathy fails to address the underlying issue and thus puts the patient at risk. Critics feel that the homeopathic principle of "like cures like" is problematic given that a particular symptom can be caused by so many different processes. Chest pain could be caused by acid reflux, a pulled muscle, bronchitis, or a heart attack: It is questioned how the treatment for all of these could be the same. It doesn't make sense to many scientists that one could take a substance that causes chest pain, dilute it until no molecule of it remains, spray the resultant liquid on a sugar pill, and use this to treat many different diseases that can induce chest pain.

- When being prepared, homeopathic remedies are diluted many times over, often to the point that not even one molecule of the remedy substance is still present in the final product. Proponents of homeopathy feel that even when there is no longer any trace of the remedy substance in a homeopathic preparation, the water "remembers," or has been affected in some way by, the substance that was once present.

  Skeptics feel that if that were true, the water would also "remember" everything else that had ever touched it over the millennia. They find it difficult to understand how the water "knows" which of the many substances it has at some point come into contact with is the one that is intended as a remedy. It has also been pointed out that although there may not be one single molecule of the original remedy present in a homeopathic product, there are certain to be many other molecules, such as those from dust, pollen, insect parts, skin cells, and so on; it is hard for scientists to imagine how a homeopathic substance that is no longer detectable in the solution would somehow be more active than those that are actually present.

Most studies of homeopathy in humans have focused on determining whether the remedies have any more effect than a placebo. Because the placebo effect is very powerful, real reduction in symptoms can occur if patients believe they are receiving a useful therapy. You might assume that the effects of placebos are all imaginary, but although a patient's impression of symptoms can be subjective, placebos can also have a tangible effect. For example, by reducing a patient's stress level, a placebo may lower blood pressure or boost immune function.

There have been several large-scale studies undertaken to compare the results of homeopathy with those of placebos. These have generally been carried out by analyzing a number of homeopathic trials and summarizing the results. The authors of these large studies compile many research trials, select those that have been properly conducted (using adequate randomization, blinding, and so on), and then perform statistical analysis. One hindrance has been the fact that many homeopathic trials have not been well designed, based on the principles I discussed at the beginning of the chapter.

Many of the trials regarding homeopathy, for example, resemble our initial theoretical experiment examining the benefits of vitamin E for itchy dogs, in which we simply gave vitamin E to one group of dogs, who eventually stopped scratching. Many homeopathic trials involve a small number of individuals who are given a homeopathic remedy, without any randomization and lacking a control group receiving a placebo or another type of treatment. With this method, it is not even possible to eliminate the effect of the researchers' own bias, especially when the assessed results are subjective, such as an inflamed area appearing less red or swollen. In order to fully and adequately investigate the usefulness of homeopathy for various conditions, well-conducted future research will be extremely helpful.

Evidence Regarding Homeopathy in Dogs and Cats

There has been very little published research on the use of homeopathy in pets. I was able to find one blinded, placebo-controlled study on the use of an available homeopathic remedy for skin allergies in dogs. This trial did not find any benefit of the remedy.

Risks of Homeopathy

Ironically, the same questions that are relevant to the effectiveness of homeopathy also apply to the possibility of risks. If the skeptics are correct, and the extremely diluted nature of homeopathic remedies renders them useless, then there should also be no risk to taking them. If homeopathic remedies do indeed have some activity that is not currently scientifically explainable, then we also cannot yet say what the risks may be to our pets, given how little research has been done in this area. Since this activity has not been well explored in dogs or cats, it is not possible to assess any possible harm that could arise. In theory, it is hard to imagine any toxicity from such diluted preparations, but if there is an effect we do not yet understand, this effect must be further evaluated before safety can be determined.

If an unproven homeopathic remedy is used in place of proven conventional therapy for a serious health issue, then the risk is of the animal potentially succumbing to the disease due to ineffective treatment.

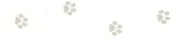

There are many additional, smaller branches of alternative veterinary medicine. An in-depth discussion of the history, methods, and evidence regarding each one would require its own book. None of these areas has yet been fully investigated in animals, and all are therefore considered to be experimental when used in pets. You can find definitions and descriptions of various approaches at the website of the National Center for Complementary and Alternative Medicine, www.nccam.nih.gov/health.

At this point, we are a long way from safe, educated use of any alternative medical approach for dogs and cats. These fields are yet to be fully explored even in human medicine—adequate well-performed clinical trials have not yet been carried out. Little by little, this is starting to occur. In veterinary medicine, there has been very little organized investigation in the alternative fields; we have skipped straight to administering these treatments without first performing due diligence to ensure we are using safe and effective therapy. Although this approach is tempting, since natural-sounding modalities are appealing—and whenever a pet is ill, we tend to become more venturesome in our quest for aid—we must be very careful not to risk harming the pets we are seeking to protect.

If you are considering the use of alternative medicine for your pet, this chapter is just a starting point. You should fully and objectively evaluate any approach you are contemplating, just as you are doing for veterinary medicine as a whole by reading this book. The NCCAM website above is a good general resource. You will also want to do additional reading, and investigate the scientific evidence for yourself. The website www. veterinarywatch.com has links to much of the veterinary and human scientific literature in this area.

The more educated you become, the better job you can do of caring for your pet, and the less subject you will be to the opinions of others. Be aware that there is much heated controversy in this area; this is why I choose to evaluate the evidence for myself, and so should you. While others may have a personal stake in defending one or another point of view, my only goal, and I hope yours, is to make the most informed decisions possible in order to best protect and care for animals.

COMPLEMENTARY AND ALTERNATIVE MEDICINE: WORKSHEET

If you are considering the use of complementary or alternative medicine for your pet, you can use the following list as an aid.

- Always treat your pet under the guidance of a licensed, reputable veterinarian.

- Evaluate any veterinary practice you frequent using the standards discussed in chapter 1.

- Be sure to ask your veterinarian before giving any herbs, supplements, or other substances to your pet.

- When questions arise regarding ingredient safety, contact the ASPCA's Animal Poison Control Center (888-426-4435) or another reputable animal poison control resource for safety information.

- Be extremely cautious about using herbs or supplements if your pet takes other medication. Investigate possible interactions and speak with your veterinarian.

- If your pet may have surgery or another procedure, be sure he's not on any herbs or supplements that could alter the effects of sedatives, anesthetics, or pain medications, or could increase the risk of bleeding. Discuss this with your veterinarian.

- If your pet is ill, do not substitute alternative therapy for proven conventional treatment.

- If your pet has a serious condition that is not responding to treatment, discuss with your general veterinarian the option of referral to the relevant specialist for a consultation (see chapter 4).

CHAPTER 7

Rover on 'Roids (and Tabby, Too):

The Use and Misuse of Steroids in Veterinary Medicine

One Saturday afternoon, I received an e-mail from a worried dog owner. She needed help with her American pit bull terrier, Spike. She had adopted Spike as a stray, and although he initially seemed fine, he soon developed severe anemia, requiring multiple blood transfusions. Spike had a type of anemia called hemolytic anemia, in which the dog's red blood cells rupture within the bloodstream.

Hemolytic anemia has many possible causes, from ingested toxins that cause the red blood cells to rupture (one example is zinc, which is found in pennies), to blood parasites that damage the cells, and autoimmune disease, in which the body's own immune system mistakenly begins attacking the red blood cells. (Yes, our immune systems can make mistakes!) Because autoimmune disease is a common cause of hemolytic anemia in dogs, it had been presumed that this was the reason for the anemia in Spike's case. He had therefore been treated with high doses of corticosteroids, which are cortisone-type steroid medications. When an animal's own immune system is attacking the cells, corticosteroids are often given because these drugs strongly suppress the immune system. In this situation, corticosteroids help prevent the destruction of the red blood cells by curbing the animal's overactive immune system.

When Spike's owner contacted me, her dog had already been treated with corticosteroids for several months. The side effects of this medication had caused his muscles to waste away, and he had developed a severe fungal infection of his lungs, heart, and skin due to the prolonged suppression of his immune system. He was still anemic as well, and his owner was very concerned about Spike's chance of survival.

When I read Spike's story, I wondered if he might be suffering from a blood parasite rather than autoimmune disease. It has come to light over the past few years that American pit bull terriers are frequently infected by a canine blood parasite called *Babesia gibsoni*. This tiny organism causes anemia by damaging the dog's red blood cells, and is likely passed from dog to dog by biting, even in play. It may also be passed from the mother dog straight to her puppies. Based on his breed and symptoms, there was a good chance that Spike was infected with *Babesia,* and if this was in fact the case, the corticosteroids were likely making matters worse by weakening Spike's immune system.

When Spike was tested for *Babesia,* the results showed that he was indeed infected with this parasite. It was amazing to me, and a testament to Spike's spirit and his owner's determination, that he had survived this long with the infection untreated and with his immune system so compromised.

Now the challenge was for Spike to hang in there long enough for the *Babesia* medication to have a chance to work, and for the effects of the corticosteroids to finally wear off. Because his immune system had been weakened by the months of corticosteroids, it was a long, hard battle for Spike to conquer the microscopic parasite he harbored in his body. He also required aggressive treatment for the life-threatening fungal infection he had acquired. In the end, Spike's strength and spirit, and his owner's devotion, carried the day, and he did indeed win his battle with *Babesia.*

There are too many examples of the hazards of the overzealous use of corticosteroids. An elderly cat named Simon is another one who comes to mind. Simon's owner had noticed that the cat's gums were very red, and that his mouth seemed painful. At that time, he was eating normally and appeared to be feeling fine, but she was worried about what was going on in his mouth. She took the cat to her neighborhood veterinary practice, where he was given several injections and sent home on a liquid medication. Since then, Simon's health had gone quickly downhill; he had developed severe nasal congestion and a thick, yellow discharge from his nose. He had then lost his appetite, not surprising since he was feeling miserable and he probably couldn't smell anything. Simon had now lost a lot of weight and was progressively weakening; at this point his owner was attempting to force food into him without much success. She was still giving him the liquid medication.

On the day Simon was seen at the veterinarian's office, the injections he received were both corticosteroids: one a very long-acting product, and the other more short-acting. The liquid medication he was sent home with contained yet another corticosteroid. The cat's immune system was being completely suppressed—no wonder he had a respiratory infection! Unfortunately, with the long-acting steroid in his system, which would last for weeks to months, things were unlikely to get better anytime soon.

Most feline respiratory infections are viral, and antibiotics can only help by combating any secondary bacterial infection; the cat's own immune system has to fight the virus, and the steroids were preventing Simon's immune system from doing this. And without help from his immune system, antibiotics wouldn't be able to take care of a bacterial infection, either. Like many cats, Simon had probably had a cold caused by a feline herpesvirus at some point during his life, and just as herpes does in humans, feline herpes remains in the cat's body forever. When he received all the steroids, his immune system was weakened, and the herpes flared up and took hold. He had probably originally had gingivitis (inflamed gums from dental problems), which is common in older cats, and now on top of that he had a severe viral respiratory infection that he couldn't fight off.

Unfortunately, Simon did not win his battle. With his immune system sabotaged by the corticosteroids he had received, he simply did not have the strength at his age to withstand the combined effects of the respiratory infection, the gingivitis, and his subsequent loss of appetite. Although his family made a valiant effort to pull him through, in the end they could not stand to watch him struggle as days went on without signs of improvement, and they finally made the decision to let him go.

Spike and Simon were both victims of one of the most common pitfalls in veterinary medicine: the overuse of steroid medications. This may sound like something that happens in the world of professional sports, but I'm not talking about the kind of anabolic steroids that athletes use. I am referring to what are called corticosteroids, or cortisone-type steroid medications that come in many forms. In this chapter, I'll discuss the proper and improper use of corticosteroids, and how vigilant pet owners can guard against the inappropriate use of these drugs on their pets.

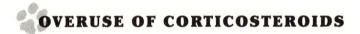OVERUSE OF CORTICOSTEROIDS

One of the most notorious issues in the practice of veterinary medicine is the overuse of corticosteroid medications. Many veterinarians are frustrated by what they feel is the misuse of these drugs by some in the profession. There are without doubt health conditions in animals for which treatment with corticosteroids is clearly indicated, but these powerful drugs are sometimes used as a panacea for whatever symptom the pet's owner complains of, and often to the patient's ultimate detriment. It is important for pet owners to be aware of the proper use of corticosteroids, so they can protect their pets while understanding that corticosteroids can serve a very useful role in certain situations.

What are corticosteroids?

Corticosteroids, also called glucocorticoids, are medications related to the natural hormone called cortisol, a steroid hormone that the body normally produces in minute amounts. There are many different preparations of corticosteroid medications, from short-, intermediate-, or long-acting injections, to pills and liquids of different types and strengths, and also topical creams and ointments. You can often recognize these medications by the letters *-one* at the end of the name: prednisone, dexamethasone, hydrocortisone, and so on. However, the brand names will not have this telltale suffix. Some brands of corticosteroid medications include the letters *cort* somewhere in the name.

Corticosteroids have effects on essentially every cell and system in the body. The most important effects for you to know about are:

- Suppression of the immune system.

- Resistance to insulin.

- Thinning of the skin and decreased healing capability.

- Increased acid in the gastrointestinal system along with decreased production of the cells that line the stomach and intestines.

- Decreased intestinal absorption of calcium and increased absorption of fat.

- Increased fat and cholesterol in the blood.

- Decreased bone growth and osteoporosis.

- Liver damage.

- Muscular weakness.

- Fluid retention.

- Poor hair growth.

What does this mean for my pet?

Let's look at some of these issues one by one, and discuss how they could actually affect your pet.

Suppression of the Immune System

Most of the time, when corticosteroids are used by veterinarians, this is the effect that is being sought. This may sound odd, as we know that we need our immune systems to work well for us to be healthy, but suppressing the immune system will also decrease inflammation anywhere in the body, and many symptoms in pets are caused by inflammation. For example, a dog with itchy skin from allergies has inflammation of the skin, so corticosteroids will decrease the itchiness. A cat who is coughing from asthma has inflammation of the bronchial tubes, so corticosteroids will decrease the coughing. You've seen this anti-inflammatory effect yourself when you've used cortisone cream for a skin rash.

In fact, infections also often cause inflammation, so corticosteroids may temporarily decrease the symptoms of an infection even while they are making it difficult for the body to battle it by suppressing the immune system. This effect can sometimes trick us into thinking that corticosteroids are solving the problem when in some situations they are just masking the symptoms. Because of this temporary lessening of symptoms, it can be very tempting to use corticosteroids to make a sick animal feel better, rather than to search for the underlying cause of the animal's condition. This shortcut can backfire, however—say, if the animal does have some sort of infection that will now flourish unchecked.

If only the anti-inflammatory property of corticosteroids did not come at such a high price, it would be a wonderful thing. But even when corticosteroids are used properly, they can have serious side effects, so the trick is to use them only when necessary and as sparingly as possible. In terms of the immune system, the price tag is decreased ability to fight any current infection, along with a higher susceptibility to new infections. This side effect can be very serious, or even fatal.

It is essential to be sure that the pet's symptoms are not being caused by an infection of any type before beginning treatment with corticosteroids. It is also important to monitor pets on corticosteroids for the development of new infections, which are more likely to occur in animals taking these drugs. For example, many animals on long-term corticosteroids will develop urinary tract infections.

Some autoimmune diseases are caused by the animal's own immune system attacking parts of the body, such as the blood cells or joints, and corticosteroids are an important component of the treatment regimen for these conditions. Along with other drugs that also affect the immune system, corticosteroids are used to dampen the excessive immune activity that is causing the condition.

In short, the immune-suppressive action of corticosteroids is a double-edged sword. If appropriate caution is not taken, it can be very dangerous. Still, when used carefully in the correct situations, this effect can be lifesaving.

Resistance to Insulin

Insulin is the hormone produced by the pancreas that helps us to process our blood sugar. It is responsible for the uptake of blood sugar into cells, so the sugar can be utilized by the body. A deficiency of insulin or resistance to the effects of insulin can cause diabetes, resulting in high blood sugar, sugar in the urine, "starvation" of the cells, and often ketoacidosis (a condition of dangerous acidosis in the body due to unregulated diabetes).

Because corticosteroids cause insulin resistance in the body, meaning they create a condition whereby the body cannot respond properly to insulin, their use can lead to diabetes. This seems to happen more often in cats, and is a particularly common side effect of long-acting corticosteroid injections. The diabetes caused by corticosteroids may be temporary or permanent, and requires the owner to give the animal twice-daily insulin injections. Because of the danger of diabetes, I try to avoid the use of long-acting corticosteroids.

Poor Healing, Thinning of the Skin, Hair Loss, and Poor Hair Growth

Another effect of corticosteroids, particularly if they are given for a long period of time, is thinning of the skin. In extreme cases, the skin will easily tear from normal handling, and these wounds will not heal properly. This effect can be reversed if corticosteroid administration is ceased, but in cases where the skin has begun to tear, it can take a very long time for the situation to improve.

Long-term corticosteroid use also decreases the animal's ability to heal, for example after an operation or injury. It can be more risky for an animal on corticosteroids to have surgery, since the tissues may not heal well and the surgical incisions can reopen. Animals on corticosteroids for long periods of time may begin balding to some degree, particularly dogs, and after the hair coat is shaved or clipped it will fail to grow back normally.

Increased Acid Production and Decreased Growth of New Cells in the Gastrointestinal System

Because of these effects, corticosteroids can cause ulcers in the stomach or intestines. These ulcers can lead to vomiting, diarrhea, blood loss, or even fatal perforation of the gastrointestinal system. For this reason, corticosteroids should *never* be given at the same time as nonsteroidal anti-inflammatory drugs (NSAIDs), which also increase the risk of ulceration. The higher the dose of corticosteroids, the more likely these side effects will occur.

Decreased Intestinal Absorption of Calcium, Increased Calcium Loss, and Decreased Bone Growth

Through a number of mechanisms, long-term use of corticosteroids can lead to osteoporosis. (This fact seems to result in more problems for humans than pets.) Additionally, the increased loss of calcium into the urine may cause calcium-based stones to form in the urinary tract, and corticosteroids can also lead to calcium deposition in various tissues in the body. For example, in a condition called calcinosis cutis, calcium deposits form in the skin, causing the pet much discomfort.

Liver Damage

Corticosteroids cause an increase on blood tests of a liver enzyme called serum alkaline phosphatase, or SAP. This change occurs in dogs but not cats, and is generally reversible when corticosteroids are stopped; in high doses or over a period of time, however, corticosteroids can cause serious liver problems. An elevated SAP enzyme is expected in a dog on corticosteroids and generally no cause for alarm, but if the dog becomes jaundiced or has other evidence of liver dysfunction, the drugs may need to be decreased or discontinued.

Fluid Retention

This side effect is most relevant in pets who have a preexisting heart condition. In pets who have a leaky heart valve, thickened heart muscle, or other heart problems (which sometimes, but not always, can be detected by listening for a heart murmur), the fluid retention caused by corticosteroids can cause the animal to go into congestive heart failure. Corticosteroids must be used very cautiously in pets who are suspected of having any type of heart condition.

🐾 PROPER USE OF CORTICOSTEROIDS

When treated with respect, corticosteroids are a very useful component of treatment for a number of diseases. However, a few important principles should be followed to minimize complications and ensure that these powerful drugs are only used when truly indicated.

A diagnosis should be made** prior **to corticosteroid administration: Using corticosteroids without a diagnosis may hinder identification of a problem or even make it worse. Corticosteroids can delay proper diagnosis by temporarily alleviating symptoms, and may actually make diagnosis of many diseases much more difficult or even impossible. Because corticosteroids can change the results of medical tests, it is essential to complete all diagnostics before treating a pet with corticosteroids. For accurate results, any blood tests, X-rays, biopsies, ultrasound exam, or other advanced procedures should be done before corticosteroids are given if possible.

For example, if an animal is suspected of having a condition of the gastrointestinal tract called inflammatory bowel disease (a common problem in pets), treatment with corticosteroids before intestinal samples are taken will change the appearance of the biopsies so that the laboratory examining the tissue may be unable to make a correct analysis. This is even more of an issue with certain kinds of cancer. In these cases, administration of corticosteroids before all diagnostic testing is complete can make the cancer invisible, thus delaying diagnosis and treatment—sometimes for months.

Corticosteroids shouldn't be used as a catchall treatment for a variety of symptoms, especially in the absence of a diagnosis. This is a trap that veterinarians may fall into, often because they feel that pet owners want a quick fix, and corticosteroids will lessen many symptoms temporarily. Without a diagnosis, however, this quick fix has not solved the problem, only briefly alleviated the symptoms, and in some cases it could even exacerbate the underlying condition. For example, an animal with a common kind of cancer called lymphoma may have enlarged lymph nodes, and corticosteroids will cause the abnormal lymph nodes to temporarily shrink. The cancer is still present, but it will now go undiagnosed for much longer and may also become more resistant to treatment due to the prior treatment with corticosteroids.

The Story of Mia

I remember one cat, Mia, I met during my residency program. She was sent to me because she had developed difficulty breathing due to fluid around her lungs. Her veterinarian had taken a sample of the fluid, and then given her a corticosteroid injection. When I saw the cat, she was still having trouble breathing, so I removed the remaining fluid from her chest cavity. I submitted both fluid samples (the first veterinarian's sample taken before the corticosteroids were given, and my sample taken several hours later) to the laboratory for analysis. The results showed many lymphoma cancer cells in the first sample, but none in the second; that is how quickly corticosteroids can "hide" cancer and affect test results. If this cat had been given corticosteroids before any fluid sample was taken, we would have been unable to diagnose her cancer.

Of course, another major concern if the animal's condition is not definitively diagnosed before corticosteroids are given is that if the problem turns out to be an infection, the animal may become much sicker due to suppression of the immune system. Spike's case was a good example: By weakening his natural immune system, the corticosteroids given to him allowed the blood parasite *Babesia* he was carrying to flourish.

Long-acting corticosteroids should be avoided if possible: As I discussed earlier, there are many types of corticosteroids on the market, including a very long-acting injection with effects lasting weeks or even months. We see many more side effects with this long-acting injection, one of the most common being diabetes. Long-acting steroid injections have also been associated with the development of a kind of tumor called a fibrosarcoma. Although veterinarians and pet owners may find it convenient to use this long-acting preparation, it must be carefully considered in each case whether the benefits outweigh the risk of serious side effects.

One of the few indications for using this type of injection is a pet who truly needs long-term corticosteroid therapy (based on a firm diagnosis), and who cannot be medicated in any other way. Given the plethora of routes that oral medications can be given these days, including pills, flavored liquids, flavored pill pockets, and even medication formulated into treats, this situation should rarely arise.

TIP Several companies now offer pill pockets to help owners medicate their pets. These pill pockets are hollow, flavored treats in which a tablet or capsule can be hidden. Many of my clients have found these to be wonderfully helpful.

Other therapies should be tried first when appropriate: For some disease processes, corticosteroids are the mainstay of treatment, and although combination therapy with other medications may decrease the dose or duration of corticosteroid therapy that is needed, their use cannot be avoided.

For other conditions, though, there are alternative treatment options that can be tried before turning to corticosteroids. For example, a dog with allergic skin disease could be treated with antihistamines and a hypoallergenic diet, or could see a dermatologist for allergy testing and injections. Consultation with the relevant specialist for the pet's condition may be helpful in formulating treatment regimens that minimize or avoid the use of corticosteroids.

The animal should be closely monitored for side effects, and the corti-corticosteroid dose adjusted accordingly: The effects of corticosteroids vary from individual to individual. Side effects that are visible to pet owners can include increased thirst and urination, hunger, panting in dogs, muscle weakness and loss, and thinning of the skin and hair coat. These side effects are generally much more apparent in dogs; in fact, if a cat on corticosteroids seems significantly more thirsty, the cat should be tested for diabetes immediately.

When corticosteroids are truly needed, some degree of side effects must be anticipated and accepted; however, if side effects are excessive, dose adjustment should be considered. In my experience, the most extreme side effects are seen in larger dogs, who may receive too high a dose if the calculation is based solely on body weight. Most medications used by veterinarians are dosed by the animal's body weight in pounds or kilograms. But powerful medications with life-threatening side effects, such as chemotherapy or corticosteroids, should often be dosed according to another measurement, meters squared, which calculates the animal's body-surface area. This method allows the dose to be more precisely tailored to the animal's individual metabolism and helps to avoid overdose.

If you have a medium- to large-sized dog being treated with corticosteroids, you may want to ask the veterinarian to calculate the dose based on your dog's size in meters squared rather than body weight, in order to lessen the side effects he will suffer. If alarming effects such as severe panting, muscle wasting of the head so that the shape of the skull bones is visible through the skin, the need to urinate constantly, or incessant thirst are noted, the dose may be excessive.

The animal should be evaluated for any individual issues that may predispose her to more severe side effects of corticosteroid treatment: Animals with certain conditions or characteristics may be more likely to experience serious side effects when treated with corticosteroids. These are a few examples:

- As I discussed above, animals with heart conditions may develop congestive heart failure if given corticosteroids. The dose should be adjusted accordingly, and the patient monitored carefully.

- Overweight animals, particularly obese cats, are more likely to become diabetic when treated with corticosteroids. Animals who are already diabetic may experience worsening of their diabetes.

- Since corticosteroids may lead to inflammation of the pancreas, they should be used cautiously in animals who have suffered from an inflamed pancreas (pancreatitis) in the past.

- Animals who are currently being treated with nonsteroidal anti-inflammatory medications (NSAIDs)—for arthritis, say—should not be given corticosteroids until the NSAIDs have been discontinued and are completely out of the animal's system. This is because both types of drugs can cause gastrointestinal ulceration, and the additive effect would put the animal at extreme risk.

- Animals must be carefully evaluated for infections of any type before being treated with corticosteroids, since these drugs will weaken the animal's immune system. There are a few situations where certain types of infections may set off an exaggerated response by the immune system, requiring cautious use of corticosteroids during treatment for the infection, but this is relatively rare.

- Animals who will be having surgery may have more difficulty healing if they are being treated with corticosteroids. If possible, the use of corticosteroids should be avoided before surgery is performed and the animal has fully healed.

CONDITIONS FOR WHICH CORTICOSTEROIDS SHOULD BE USED

For certain conditions, corticosteroids are very helpful. I have listed just some examples below. Keep in mind that, if possible, corticosteroids should not be used until every effort has been made to definitively diagnose the condition.

Autoimmune Diseases

These are conditions in which the animal's own immune system attacks some part of the body. They are also called immune-mediated diseases.

For example, the immune system may attack the blood cells (red cells, white cells, or platelet cells), joints, muscles, skin, or organs. There are many forms of autoimmune disease: hemolytic anemia, rheumatoid arthritis, autoimmune skin diseases, and more.

Generally, when a pet is being treated for autoimmune disease with corticosteroids, a high dose is used for the first two to four weeks, and the dose is slowly lowered over several months as the animal's condition improves. For example, the animal may be given the medication twice a day for a month, then once a day for a month, and so on. The side effects will be at their worst during the initial period, and then will lessen as the dose is decreased. If the dose of corticosteroids is lowered too quickly, there is a higher risk of relapse, so patience is required. Often additional medications that also suppress the immune system are used in order to minimize the dose of corticosteroids that is required.

Inflammatory Bowel Disease

Inflammatory bowel disease, a condition in which the intestines become inflamed due to an overactive immune response (sometimes against particular food proteins), causes symptoms such as weight loss, diarrhea, or vomiting. It is diagnosed with intestinal biopsies obtained via endoscopy, laparoscopy, or surgery (see chapter 5). Corticosteroids are often used as one component of treatment, along with prescription diets and sometimes other types of medication.

Some patients with inflammatory bowel disease can be gradually taken off medication after several months of treatment, although others require long-term corticosteroid therapy. Generally, the corticosteroid dose is slowly tapered down if possible, much like the treatment of autoimmune disease described above.

Feline Asthma

Cats can develop asthma similar to that seen in humans. For long-term treatment, we now use inhaled corticosteroids to treat the problem locally in the lungs, thus avoiding side effects elsewhere in the body. Before the development of inhaled medication for asthmatic cats, many of these patients became diabetic due to the frequent use of oral or injected corticosteroids.

Asthma in Cats

Feline asthma causes symptoms such as coughing, panting, and difficulty breathing. When cats cough, owners often confuse it with a hair ball, since a cat's cough does not sound like a person's. Because of this, many asthmatic cats go undiagnosed until they have a crisis or develop severe lung damage. On the other hand, cats with noisy nasal breathing—for example, due to a prior viral infection in the nose or obesity—are sometimes erroneously labeled as asthmatic, since their breathing may sound wheezy. However, the wheezy sound in this case is actually coming from the nose, which is not typical of asthma.

There are several excellent websites for owners of cats with asthma. One is www.fritzthebrave.com, which offers useful advice including the suggested protocol for the use of inhaled steroids. The mask that's used to administer the medication to cats can be ordered at www.aerokat.com. The medication itself requires a prescription from a veterinarian.

It is very important that cats with asthma are not exposed to cigarette smoke, and in fact it appears that many cases of feline asthma are caused by secondhand smoke in the household. For cat owners who smoke, maybe this is the incentive you need to finally quit!

Certain Types of Cancer

Some kinds of cancer are treated with corticosteroids, generally along with other medications such as chemotherapy. Examples are lymphoma, myeloma, and some mast cell tumors. Corticosteroids can actually kill certain types of cancer cells and may shrink some tumors. However, this effect is generally not long-lasting. If a pet has symptoms that may point to cancer, such as enlarged lymph nodes or unexplained weight loss, it is imperative that a firm diagnosis is reached before any corticosteroids are given, as corticosteroids can falsify test results and also cause the cancer to be more difficult to treat successfully.

Addison's Disease

Addison's disease, also called hypoadrenocorticism, is a condition in which the adrenal glands produce insufficient amounts of certain hormones. Since these substances are required to sustain life, the animal must be continuously medicated with hormone supplements including small doses of corticosteroids. Addison's disease is seen most commonly in certain dog breeds, such as standard poodles, but can occur in any animal. Symptoms can include poor appetite, intermittent diarrhea, vomiting, weakness, and collapse. This condition is diagnosed with a blood test that measures the animal's blood cortisol level after an injection has been given to stimulate the adrenal glands to produce the hormone. If the animal has Addison's disease, the blood cortisol level will be very low.

This information about corticosteroids should not frighten you away from allowing them to be used for your pet when appropriate. Although corticosteroids should be used only in certain situations, and then with proper caution and respect, they are powerful and effective drugs for some conditions. My goal is to educate you regarding these medications so that you can help ensure that they are given to your pet only when truly indicated.

Unfortunately, pets are sometimes treated with corticosteroids without the informed consent of their owners. A corticosteroid injection may be given before the owner even realizes what is happening or what the injection contains. Don't feel hesitant about asking your veterinarian to fully explain *any* medication that is being given to your pet. If you are uncomfortable with the explanation, you can ask for more details or even seek a second opinion. In the case of corticosteroids, you should feel that they are being used in a well-thought-out and fully justified manner, based on a diagnosis rather than simply as a quick, temporary fix for your pet's symptoms. Since even one dose of corticosteroids can have long-range consequences, don't be afraid to use your knowledge to protect your pet.

SAFE USE OF CORTICOSTEROIDS IN PETS: WORKSHEET

The following criteria should be met, if possible, before corticosteroids are administered to your pet. You may want to go over this list with your veterinarian if it has been suggested that your pet be given corticosteroids.

- Has your pet's condition been definitively diagnosed?

- Have all necessary tests been performed?

- Has the possibility of an infection been ruled out? (In some cases, corticosteroids may be administered simultaneously with treatment of an infection.)

- Has your pet been evaluated for any conditions that may increase the risk of side effects of corticosteroids, such as a heart condition, diabetes, or obesity?

- Have any appropriate alternative treatments for the condition been considered or attempted?

- Could consultation with a specialist potentially offer other options?

- Is the corticosteroid that will be used the safest one for this situation?

- If a long-acting injection is being considered, is it absolutely necessary?

During treatment with corticosteroids, the following monitoring should be in place:

- The pet should be monitored for the development of unacceptable levels of side effects, and the dose adjusted if necessary.

- The pet should be monitored for the development of any secondary infections, one of the most common being infection of the urinary tract.

- The pet should be monitored for the development of any symptoms that might indicate the onset of diabetes, and the blood or urine sugar checked if necessary.

- If the pet fails to respond to corticosteroid therapy, an alternative diagnosis or treatment should be considered.

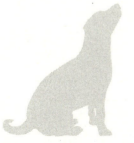

Pet Peeves:
Where to Turn If Things Go Wrong

The goal of this book is to aid you in ensuring that your pet always receives a high standard of health care. By teaching you how to choose the best veterinary practice for your pet, how to evaluate the medical care your pet is receiving, and about the resources that are available for animals in need of advanced diagnostics or specialized treatment, I hope to help you avoid situations in which you feel that your pet did not receive appropriate care. The ideal strategy is to safeguard your pet proactively by being an informed guardian.

However, inevitably there are instances when an owner becomes concerned that a pet received inadequate care or that a mistake may have occurred. When this type of concern arises, what should the pet owner do? How can pet owners know if their worries are valid, and what recourses are available if their pet has indeed been harmed?

SEPARATING GRIEF FROM BLAME

It's important to realize that when a pet becomes ill or dies, it is a natural reaction to cast about for something or someone to blame. It's instinctive to seek the reasons for events. We may blame ourselves, wondering if things might have turned out differently if we had been paying closer attention to a pet's symptoms, or if we'd brought the animal to the veterinarian sooner. Or we may turn our grief outward and feel the urge to blame someone else, with the veterinarian being one obvious choice.

No matter how rational we try to be, it's hard to avoid wondering why something bad had to happen. When my ninety-two-year-old grandmother whom I adored suddenly died, I was devastated. I worried about all the things that perhaps could have been done differently. Maybe I should have done a better job of overseeing her medical care. Perhaps if the ambulance had come sooner, she might have lived. I constantly reviewed the list of what-ifs in my mind: What if she had seen a different doctor or specialist? What if she had lived in an area where the hospital was not as far away? Could the paramedics have done more? Would help have come faster if she had called 911 instead of using the medical alert service I had installed for her? Of course with time, some logical part of me had to admit that these thoughts were somewhat irrational, and that it is not exactly unexpected for a ninety-two-year-old to pass away.

It's very hard for us to accept that sometimes sad things just happen. They don't have to be anybody's fault, and they are often unavoidable. If you find yourself struggling with these kinds of emotions about a pet's illness or death, try to separate your immediate reactions from your more rational side. If you are inclined to place responsibility on the veterinarian or practice, wait until you feel calmer and then make an attempt to review the facts in an orderly fashion. Is there truly a reason to suspect that negligence occurred, or are you just very upset about your pet and angry at the world? You may find it helpful to discuss the situation with an objective friend.

Remember also that medicine is not an exact science. It requires a fallible human being to use clues to decipher a mystery: What is wrong with this patient and what is the best treatment? Unfortunately, even with our best efforts, doctors do not always succeed. Some medical cases are particularly confusing, and with hindsight we realize that a different diagnosis or treatment might have been possible. This can be hard for a pet owner to face, but does not necessarily mean that the veterinarian should be held responsible. We'll talk in the next section about some relatively objective measures to help you decide if your pet's care was appropriate.

Additionally, financial considerations often play a part in pet owners' feelings of frustration. It can be difficult to accept the simultaneous loss of a pet with payment of a large medical bill. Pet owners sometimes feel that they shouldn't have to pay for the care of a pet who died. Of course this isn't the way medicine works; if the veterinarian and the practice staff did their best to help an animal who succumbed to an illness, they should be compensated for their time and services.

EVALUATING YOUR PET'S CARE

Let's talk about some criteria that may help you to make an initial, general assessment of whether your pet received appropriate care. For a deeper analysis and more subtle medical questions, you will need the help of a veterinarian who is willing to review your pet's record and give a frank opinion. As I will discuss later, this help may not be easy to find. And you should recognize that another veterinarian's impressions can be somewhat subjective: Two doctors may not necessarily agree on the best course of action for a particular patient. It's important that the reviewing veterinarian is able to support her opinions with references or other evidence.

It is also essential that the reviewing veterinarian have access to the complete medical records rather than just your account of events. I have seen many cases in which a simple misunderstanding or breakdown in communication caused even well-informed owners to draw inaccurate conclusions about their pets' care. In these cases, the reviewing veterinarian was able to put the owners' mind at ease simply by reading through the records and clearing up the confusion.

When making an effort to objectively evaluate your pet's care, here are some useful parameters to consider:

1. Are the medical records proper and complete?

In the first chapter, we discussed the qualities of an appropriate medical record. You can use these guidelines to evaluate your pet's file. You are entitled to a copy of your pet's *complete* record. The copy should be of every page of the record, not selected ones. If you are concerned that you may not receive the entire file or that it may be altered, visit the practice in person. First, politely request to review your pet's original record, so you can make note of the number and appearance of the pages. Then ask for a copy, indicate that you are willing to wait for this to be made, and be patient until the receptionist has time to address your request. It may not be possible for a busy practice to make you a copy the same day, in which case you can review the record and then return for the copy.

These are the record components we discussed in the first chapter with some additional detail:

- Each time your pet was seen, a thorough medical history and complete physical exam should be recorded. See chapter 2 for a full explanation of these items.

- If your pet had surgery, the record should include a surgery report, which is a complete description of the operation or procedure. The veterinarian should record how the surgery was performed step by step, what kind of suture material was chosen, and which suturing technique was used. There should also be a clear record of the anesthesia that your pet received, with notations of her vital signs, such as the heart rate and blood oxygen level, throughout the procedure.

- If your pet received medication, the record should clearly note the name of the medication, how much was dispensed, and for how long it was to be given.

- If your pet was hospitalized, the record should include daily treatment sheets with all fluids and medications given each day, including doses and routes of administration. If you are not sure what your animal received and want to make certain that everything was properly recorded, it may help to compare the record with your itemized bill.

- For hospitalized patients, a daily physical examination, notes on the patient's progress, and the doctor's plan should be recorded *each day*.

- All test results should be included, blood tests and results of other diagnostics such as X-rays or ultrasound examination.

- If your pet was admitted to the hospital, there should be a copy of the financial estimate that you were given at the outset.

2. Did your pet receive adequate nursing care?

Sometimes pet owners feel as though their pet might have suffered harm due to being left alone for too long or by improper nursing care. If you have such concerns, these are some questions to consider.

- If your pet was hospitalized for serious illness or major surgery, was there an overnight and weekend technician or doctor at the practice with your pet? If not, were you offered the option of transferring your pet to a facility that could provide twenty-four-hour care if one exists in your area?

- If veterinary technicians administered medication, anesthesia, or other treatments to your pet, were the technicians properly licensed or registered if your state's laws require it? You can check if your state requires veterinary technicians to be licensed by contacting the state licensing board.

3. Were any advanced diagnostic tests that were done on your pet performed by an individual with adequate qualifications?

Another concern often raised by pet owners is whether a pet's condition was properly diagnosed. Some pets undergo advanced diagnostic procedures as part of the investigation into the cause of their illness, and owners may question the validity of the results.

- If your pet received advanced diagnostics such as an ultrasound exam or endoscopy, did the person who performed the test have the proper training and experience? See chapter 5 for a detailed discussion of this issue. Currently, there is no codified regulation of this area in veterinary medicine, meaning that no certification or minimal skill level is required to offer these types of services. However, if you find that the person who performed such a procedure on your pet may not have had sufficient training (such as rigorous instruction during a residency program in the relevant specialty area), this may support your concerns about the adequacy of your pet's care.

- The accuracy of test results can be evaluated by having the same procedure repeated by a highly qualified individual, another route of diagnosis appropriate for your pet's condition such as surgical exploration, or by a postmortem exam in the case of a deceased pet.

4. Were you offered referral to a veterinary specialist or advanced care facility if appropriate?

Pet owners may feel that their pets could have been better helped had they been offered the option of seeing a specialist. The situations listed below are examples of when a pet should be referred for a second opinion or intensive care. See chapter 4 for more information on specialists. These recommendations are most relevant if the pertinent specialist exists where you live; not all types of veterinary specialist can be found in every area. You can check whether there is a particular type of specialist practicing in your city or state by checking on that specialty's website. If you were offered referral and declined, the general veterinarian should have made note of this in the record.

It is important not only whether referral was offered, but also if this was done in a timely fashion. The American Veterinary Medical Association's Guidelines for Referral state: "Practitioners who determine that a second opinion is desirable or that they are unable to diagnose a condition or a disease adequately or to treat an animal appropriately, should make the client aware of other diagnostic or treatment options. This referral should be done in a timely manner relative to the health of the patient."

- The owner of a pet with any ongoing illness that the general veterinarian is having difficulty diagnosing or successfully treating should be offered referral to the appropriate veterinary specialist for consultation.

- The owner of a pet having major surgery should be offered referral to a veterinary surgeon. If a pet needs surgery that calls for intensive postoperative monitoring (such as an operation that could lead to blood loss, heart arrhythmias, or severe pain), the owner should be given the option of having it performed at a facility with twenty-four-hour care if the general veterinarian's practice does not offer this.

- The owner of a pet with a heart murmur, congestive heart failure, or another cardiac condition should be offered referral to a cardiologist.

- The owner of a pet with cancer should be offered referral to an oncologist.

- The owner of a pet with severe neurological symptoms or seizures that are difficult to control should be offered referral to a neurologist.

- The owner of a pet with serious disease or injury of the eye should be offered referral to an ophthalmologist.

- The owner of a pet with skin disease that is difficult to successfully diagnose or treat should be offered referral to a dermatologist.

- The owner of a pet with ongoing vomiting, diarrhea, weight loss, increased thirst, abnormal urination, blood work abnormalities, or other symptoms of a problem with the internal organs and systems should be offered referral to an internist if the condition persists.

5. If your pet had anesthesia, were up-to-date techniques employed, and was your pet properly monitored?

In the first chapter, I listed some ways to assess whether a veterinary practice is performing anesthesia using modern protocols and with appropriate monitoring. If you believe your pet's anesthesia might have been unsafe, you can check if these standards were followed:

- For surgery or major procedures, the practice should use modern gas anesthetics, such as isoflurane or sevoflurane.

- Animals under anesthesia should be intubated (have an oxygen tube in their trachea) and should have an intravenous catheter in place.

- During anesthesia, the pet's vital signs should be monitored by equipment such as a pulse oximeter that measures the heart rate and blood oxygen level.

RECOURSES IF YOUR PET HAS BEEN HARMED

Pet owners who after careful consideration truly feel that their pet has been harmed by a veterinarian have several potential avenues of approach. Each, however, is fraught with obstacles, which I will discuss. The four options are: a complaint to the state licensing board, a civil suit, a small-claims case, and criminal prosecution. Criminal prosecution would be appropriate if pet owners suspect that their animal was a victim of deliberate cruelty rather than negligence or veterinary malpractice. Although thankfully this situation is rare, even this can be difficult to address, since surprisingly veterinarians are exempt from the anti-cruelty laws in many states.

If you suspect abuse of an animal by anyone, including a veterinarian, this should be immediately reported to the proper authorities in your state. If you are not sure who to contact in your area, you can call the police or humane society, or look on the ASPCA's website (www.aspca.org) for help.

Let's look more closely at the two more commonly relevant options: a state board complaint or a civil lawsuit. What are the rewards and challenges that a pet owner can expect with these routes?

Filing a State Board Complaint

Every state has a veterinary medical board that oversees the licensing of veterinarians as well as other matters of professional regulation. These boards are generally composed of a group of veterinarians licensed in the state, as well as one or more members of the public. The boards review complaints by consumers against a veterinarian practicing in the state, and are responsible for taking disciplinary action if indicated. It is important to realize that state boards can only impose fines and/or suspend or revoke the veterinarian's license; they cannot compensate the pet owner financially in any way.

If you really believe that a veterinarian harmed your pet, it is essential to submit a complaint to the state board. The board must be informed by consumers if it is to effectively perform its task of protecting animals and the public. Some state boards accept complaints via e-mail; others require forms to be mailed to them. You can find the forms and other information about filing a complaint on your state board's website. The website addresses can be found at www.healthguideusa.org. Additionally, if you decide to take civil action, it will help your case if there is a state board judgment available.

It is important to realize, however, the limitations of a state board complaint against a veterinarian. As mentioned above, state boards cannot compensate pet owners financially. In addition, it is uncommon for state boards to take major disciplinary action against a veterinarian, such as license revocation. Lastly, state board proceedings can be very lengthy, and the pet owner should not wait for the results of the board complaint before deciding whether to take further action, such as a civil lawsuit. In the event that the owner does have a valid claim, this may be negated by the expiration of the statute of limitations for filing the suit if it is delayed pending the board's decision.

Bringing a Civil Lawsuit

One avenue available to pet owners is a civil lawsuit. This is a complex topic, and I will do my best to touch on the most relevant points for you. For more information, there are resources available to the interested pet owner. These are listed at the end of the chapter. The subject of veterinary malpractice liability is a controversial one, both within and outside the veterinary profession. Much of this arises from the fact that animals are currently considered to be personal property under the law.

What does it mean for pet owners that legally their pets are generally seen as property? Most important for this discussion, it means that right now in most states an owner cannot recover more than what's called the market value of their animal, no matter what the circumstances of the case. The most clear-cut case of veterinary malpractice, even one where the facts are not in dispute, could therefore in most instances result only in a negligible financial award to the owner. In fact, although pets are considered property under the law, such that a sick pet is no different than a broken appliance, they are actually in the majority of cases worth even less than most property. The truth is that most pets have almost no true financial value, if any; if you think about how many dogs and cats are euthanized in animal shelters each year, you will see what I mean. As much as we adore our pets, we would probably have a hard time giving them away.

It is often shocking to pet owners to find out that their beloved pets are considered virtually worthless property by the law, especially in light of the fact that for many people pets are like family members. This twist of the law is a holdover from the past, and although at some point the law may catch up with society, this has not yet occurred. Ironically, you probably spend more at each veterinary visit than your pet is actually "worth," so to recover any meaningful damages in a veterinary malpractice lawsuit is a challenge.

Veterinarians are thus in a strange situation. Legally, they are almost completely insulated from civil lawsuits of any consequence, since their charges are considered not patients but property. Yet they rely on the fact that many people feel far from this way about their animal companions, and instead place a high value on their pets' well-being. Of course most pet owners are not interested in the financial value of their pets but rather their emotional worth as living beings who bring joy and affection to our lives. If owners valued their pets based on the animals' market value rather than their emotional value, companion animal veterinarians would quickly go out of business. Although the current state of the law is beneficial to veterinarians, this disparity is unlikely to withstand the test of time: It is improbable that people will continue to accept the fact that they are expected to be willing to pay for whatever is best for their pets' health, and yet have little redress when things go awry.

The fact that veterinary clients are for the most part unable to successfully sue a veterinarian in any meaningful way, and that veterinary state boards are almost solely responsible for enforcing the veterinary standard of care, implies that there really isn't any independent means of ensuring that veterinarians practice high-quality medicine. The veterinary profession essentially regulates itself, and consumers have little recourse if they find this regulation lacking. Additionally, it has been argued that veterinarians' virtual immunity from significant lawsuits removes a powerful deterrent against the practice of subpar medicine. This makes it all the more essential that pet owners choose their pet's veterinarian cautiously, and proactively monitor the care their animals are receiving in an informed fashion.

Isn't anything being done to change the situation?

It has been proposed that the best solution to this dilemma, and the one that will most benefit all the parties (companion animals, the animals' human guardians, and the veterinary profession) is to pass state legislation regarding the matter. Pet owners need legal recourse when an animal is harmed, but veterinarians are understandably afraid of the consequences. Christopher Green, a lawyer who is one of the country's leading experts in this area, says, "State legislation that specifically decrees the circumstances, requirements, and limits of compensating companion animal harm would appear to be the most fair, transparent, and democratic manner of effecting any material shift in the way our legal system evaluates such loss." By passing legislation that clearly defines the relevant legal parameters, and places reasonable limits on the amount that can be awarded in a lawsuit, such legislation would hopefully answer the needs of all concerned.

Over the past several years, statutes have been introduced in multiple states to increase pet owners' potential recovery for the loss of a companion animal. However, for the most part these legislative attempts to protect pets and their owners have failed, in part because of the strong opposition of the state veterinary medical associations. A statute called the T-Bo Act (named for the sponsoring senator's dog) did pass in Tennessee in 2000, but it limits the damages an owner can collect for the death of a pet to five thousand dollars, and in any case it exempts veterinarians. Statutes introduced in other states have also made exceptions for veterinarians, so thus far the veterinary profession remains protected.

How do I proceed legally if I am convinced my pet has been wrongly harmed?

According to Laura Ireland Moore, the executive director of the National Center for Animal Law (NCAL) at Lewis & Clark Law School (www.lclark.edu/org/ncal), you should first think carefully about all the challenges you will face. Moore warns that the two biggest hurdles you will encounter initially are finding a veterinary expert witness who is willing to help you, and locating an attorney who agrees to take your case.

To bring a civil lawsuit against a veterinarian requires that another veterinarian be willing to testify. Moore notes that although you may be able to find a veterinarian to review and discuss the medical records behind the scenes, it is another matter entirely to find one who agrees to come out publicly. The best chance is often with a veterinarian who is retired or from another town, and therefore less fearful of her colleagues' disapproval. Naturally, veterinarians are reluctant to risk the disfavor of other members of their profession, even if they may privately sympathize with an animal's plight or an owner's concerns. The assistance of an expert witness may also involve a fee, and you need to be aware of this early financial outlay.

There are likely less than one hundred lawyers in the United States who take this kind of case, so it may be quite difficult to retain one in your area. You can start your search by contacting your state bar's attorney-referral network, a service every state bar offers. Some states have a category of animal law attorneys; in others you may need to find a lawyer through another related category, such as general civil law or medical malpractice. The NCAL website given above has a link to help you find an attorney in addition to links to the state bars. The NCAL also has a legal clinic that will work with a lawyer who is not very familiar with animal law, and assist her with your case.

However, be aware that you will be hampered by the fact that for a lawyer taking this type of case, the likelihood of recovering any kind of significant contingency is remote. Because of this, you will probably be charged an hourly rate, and Moore estimates that it can cost upward of fifty thousand dollars in legal fees to bring a veterinary malpractice claim! Therefore, it is important to recognize that veterinary malpractice suits don't really make economic sense for the pet owner; you must go into it with this in mind. If your goal is to recover your veterinary fees, it is probably only worth the trouble if your bills total more than ten thousand dollars.

The last hurdle you will face is the judge assigned to your case. It is a roll of the dice whether your judge will be sympathetic to the situation and willing to interpret the law in your favor. The few cases that have been successful have relied on a judge who saw the law as archaic, or perhaps was also an animal lover.

If you decide despite all of this discouraging information to press on, Moore recommends you take the following steps:

- First, if your pet is deceased, have a postmortem exam (necropsy) performed immediately. These generally must be performed within forty-eight hours or so of the animal's death, and it is important that the animal's remains have not been kept at freezing temperatures (refrigerator temperature is ideal). Most veterinary schools will perform this procedure for a fee.

- Obtain copies of all your pet's medical records, as discussed above.

- File a complaint with your state veterinary board. About two weeks after sending in the complaint, be sure to check whether the state board received it and has begun its investigation into the matter. Don't wait for the results to proceed with the next steps.

- Next, begin to track down a veterinarian who will agree to serve as an expert witness for your case. This will always be a necessity, and you will decrease your legal fees if you are prepared with an expert witness before the lawyer gets to work. You may need to look outside your geographic area, and be prepared to pay for the veterinarian's services.

- Be sure to write down everything you can think of pertaining to your pet's case, and keep meticulous records of all your conversations with the veterinary practice or other relevant parties, including dates and times.

- Once these first steps have been accomplished, you will need an attorney to take your case, and you can use the suggestions above to help you find one. Be aware that if your lawyer is inexperienced in these matters, it is unavoidable that some of your fees will go toward the time it takes for him to familiarize himself with the legal situation. The less experience he has, the more it may cost you.

Most important, be realistic. Decide before you start down this road what you are really hoping to gain. If your aim is to get to the bottom of things and find out what really happened in your pet's case, you are likely to be disappointed. Lawsuits often result in only more murkiness as things become complicated by depositions and other legal processes. If you hope that your case may help other animals or set new legal precedents that will lead to future changes, and you are fully prepared to pay the financial and emotional tolls a lawsuit can demand, perhaps you will achieve your goal.

Moore reminds us that the only way for the law to evolve and recognize the special value of our pets is through the efforts of pet lovers. Although veterinary malpractice lawsuits can be frustrating and are rarely financially rewarding, they are a potential route to change.

Small-Claims Court

If you are unable to afford a lawyer and are mainly hoping to recover your expenses, small-claims court is an option. In small-claims court, you can represent yourself, and you may be able to introduce an affidavit from your expert witness as an alternative to having the veterinarian come in to testify in person.

In small-claims court, your recovery will be limited to the money you have lost, and you will not have a chance of receiving financial compensation for your animal's sentimental value or your loss of companionship. Additionally, some malpractice cases are just too complicated for small-claims court; this option makes the most sense for fairly blatant cases (for example, an animal who had surgery on the wrong leg or a similarly obvious mistake).

Small claims is certainly a more simple and affordable route to consider if you have financial limitations, would like to minimize your investment of time and emotion, and are mainly interested in recouping your monetary losses.

USEFUL WEBSITES

- To find your state board's website address: www.healthguideusa.org.

- For help contacting your state bar, general assistance in finding a lawyer, expert advice for a lawyer inexperienced with animal law, or other information: www.lclark.edu/org/ncal.

- Information about laws pertaining to animals: www.animallaw.info.

HOW TO PROCEED IF A PET MAY HAVE BEEN HARMED: WORKSHEET

These are some steps to consider following if you are concerned your pet may have been harmed by a veterinarian.

- Calmly review the situation, objectively evaluating whether there is any concrete reason to suspect wrongdoing. Be sure that you are basing your suspicions on facts rather than emotions. Don't confuse grief with blame.

- If your pet is deceased, immediately have a postmortem exam performed—for example, at one of the veterinary schools. This will keep your options open.

- If you are uneasy about the level of care your pet received, obtain a copy of your pet's records and review them using the parameters in this book as a guide. You can also use other information you have learned here to make an educated judgment.

- Write down everything you can remember about your pet's care, including all past, present, and future conversations regarding the case.

- If you strongly feel that your pet's care was inappropriate, file a complaint with the state board immediately.

- If you may want to pursue a civil lawsuit or small-claims judgment, begin your search for a veterinarian willing to serve as an expert witness.

- If you decide to file a lawsuit and you can afford the legal fees, find a lawyer by contacting your state bar's attorney-referral network or using the NCAL website.

CHAPTER 9

Finding Peace:
Making Decisions at the End

We all sat on the kitchen floor around Dodger, petting him and telling him what a wonderful boy he was. He was such a good-hearted creature, and as sweet and gentle a dog as there could be—it had been difficult watching his inexorable physical deterioration over the past few years and more rapidly over the last couple of months. Now it had reached a point that no longer seemed fair to him.

Dodger had not been able to control his bowels for some time, and my mother-in-law, Gloria, had patiently cleaned up after him time and again. He had lost the ability to navigate stairs and other obstacles months before, but now he would often fall over when simply standing in the house, and she had found him lying in a mess unable to rise several times. What's more, he was beginning to rapidly lose weight, and I suspected that in addition to his severe arthritis he was no longer able to properly absorb nutrients from his food; in a stronger dog, I would have wanted to perform testing to investigate what was amiss with his gastrointestinal system, but for fifteen-year-old Dodger it would simply not be right to put him through any more.

As our family stroked him and murmured endearments, I gently inserted a small catheter into the vein of his hind leg. He was momentarily annoyed by the slight sting but was quickly distracted by the hands caressing his ears and relaxed. I slowly injected the sedative, feeling a lump in my throat and blinking back tears. Loving hands held his head as he fell asleep surrounded by his favorite people, and as I attached the syringe of euthanasia barbiturate to the catheter I knew that Dodger had not felt a moment's fear as he slipped away.

Gloria had already decided what she wanted to do after Dodger was gone: He would be cremated, and she would scatter his ashes in a patch of flowers in the yard where he had spent so many happy hours with the family. I knew that it was much better that she had previously settled on this plan so that in her last moments with Dodger she would not have the additional burden of having to make decisions about his remains. As we hugged her good-bye and prepared to put Dodger in the car for his final journey—to my practice, where the pet cemetery that would perform the cremation would come and get him—I could see that Gloria's heart and mind were at ease. Dodger had lived the best life a dog could ever wish for, and his end could not have been more peaceful.

For both pet and pet owner, it is essential that the last moments of an animal's life are as dignified and peaceful as possible. For the pet herself, we must minimize any pain or fear she experiences. For the pet owner, a smooth and well-handled farewell allows peace of mind and a healthy grieving process, unburdened by regret and softened by fond memories. There is of course no avoiding the heartache involved in losing a beloved pet, but the pain can be lessened if the parting is approached in a thoughtful manner.

Conversely, the stress of the situation and the trauma felt afterward will be intensified if all does not go well. An experience with my dear dog Pip taught me how important those final moments will be to the pet owner for literally years to come. I got Pip, a domineering but fiercely loyal Welsh corgi, when I was a child in middle school. Twelve years later, as I was finishing with college, Pip was losing a battle with a tumor that had started in his hard palate and spread throughout his nose and sinuses, despite several major operations to remove it.

Home from school, I found Pip fighting to breathe through his badly obstructed nasal passages. I wished he would have the sense to breathe through his mouth. At night, he would lie under my old brass bed as he always had, and it was heartbreaking to hear him struggle and wheeze. I took to sleeping on the sofa downstairs with my hand on his head, and it was clear this could not go on.

I decided that if he was going to have to be euthanized, I wanted it to be done at home. He had always been very difficult at the veterinarian's office. I had never had to do something like this before and was not sure how to proceed. I checked in the phone book and found a listing for a veterinarian who made house calls. I was scared and upset, and didn't really consider what I wanted to do with Pip after he was gone. I didn't know for sure what all my choices were, and I assumed the veterinarian would offer words of advice. I also assumed that all vets were as wonderful as those at the practice our family used for all our pets.

When the veterinarian arrived, he was grouchy and taciturn. He had come without a helper, and I had to assist him; I was shaking and felt rushed and utterly overwhelmed by the situation. The veterinarian didn't ask me what was wrong with my dog, nor did he explain the euthanasia process to me. Once he had dispatched Pip with little ceremony, he made a quick exit. When my stepfather arrived home to find me dissolved in tears, holding Pip on the sofa, he drove us to the local pet cemetery. My mother, who adored Pip, has his ashes at home to this day.

MY PHILOSOPHY

When I became a veterinarian, I remembered my experience with Pip; I still thought about it and wished I could go back and do it all differently. I never wanted a client to feel the way I had, or to be plagued by bad memories rather than comforted by happy ones. From this wish, my personal set of principles for helping owners and pets through the parting process has evolved. I think that the following guidelines should always be followed; it's sort of a pet euthanasia bill of rights.

- As a pet approaches the end of his life, whether due to illness or age, the veterinarian offers support and counsel to the pet's family members who are faced with making decisions regarding his quality of life. When appropriate, she offers referral to a specialist for a second opinion so that the pet's owners can feel confident they have explored all available treatment options. She draws on her veterinary knowledge and past experiences to help her clients understand their animal's condition and how it is likely to progress, and make informed decisions as to the most ideal timing for saying good-bye.

- As the time to let go draws near, but before the euthanasia itself, the veterinarian gently educates the owners as to the choices that will have to be made, such as what to do with the pet's remains and whether to have a postmortem exam performed, so they can consider the options beforehand. Depending on the situation, this may be days, hours, or just moments before the procedure. The clients should not feel rushed or pressured as to the best course of action; if necessary, after the euthanasia, the deceased pet is held at the practice for a day or two until they have come to a decision.

- At the time of euthanasia, the family members are given the choice of whether to stay with the pet during the process, or say good-bye and not be present. Owners should always have the option of staying with their pet if they desire.

- Just before the euthanasia, the veterinarian explains how the process will unfold, so the clients understand what is happening each step of the way. They should be prepared about what to expect, so they will not be surprised or alarmed by anything that occurs.

- A euthanasia protocol should be used that is smooth and peaceful for both the pet and the owners who are present. The drugs used should be those that offer the most tranquil transition.

- The procedure should take place in an unhurried fashion, in a quiet, private room. The family should be able to touch and speak to their pet during the entire process.

- After the procedure, the owners are offered a few moments alone with their pet if desired. Some owners may want to clip a lock of the pet's hair to keep.

If you ever feel that one of these steps is being skipped, or that you are not being offered an option that is important to you, such as to remain by your pet's side at the end, it is important to speak up. It is essential that you feel in control of the process, and that you are able to ensure your pet's comfort and your own peace of mind.

HELP WITH DECISIONS

This is a difficult topic for most of us. We naturally shy away from the concept of death and avoid talking or thinking about it most of the time. However, the fact is that most of us who love animals will face the loss of a pet at some point, or more likely several times in our lives. I believe that whatever I can do to educate pet owners and prepare them for this difficult hurdle will lessen the pain and confusion they face at the time. There are many tough decisions to be made when a pet becomes very ill or aged, and hopefully the thoughts I am sharing with you will be helpful if you find yourself in this situation.

When should a pet be euthanized? Can't pets ever die naturally?

No one knows the perfect answers to these questions, and it is really up to each of us as individuals to decide how we feel. That being said, I can offer words of guidance that have been helpful for some of my clients.

I have often thought about the concept of euthanasia for our pets. Must every pet be euthanized at some point? Should some pets be allowed to die on their own, of old age or disease? I can't answer this question for others, and for some, personal philosophical or religious considerations may come into play. I can answer only as a veterinarian who has dealt with many old and sick pets, and as a pet owner myself.

For me, it comes down to the unfortunate fact that most pets will not go comfortably in their sleep, as we might hope. Age and illness can be cruel, and I cannot bear to see an animal suffer, so I have opted for euthanasia for my pets when I felt that their discomfort was outweighing their enjoyment of life and there was absolutely nothing more I could do to help. The question that then arises for all of us is: When? How do we know when it is time to let go? These are the best answers I have been able to come up with over the years.

- The key concept is to watch for the time when the bad things in the animal's life have begun to outweigh the good things—for example, when the animal's enjoyment of your company, or his meal or walk outside, doesn't seem enough any longer to make up for whatever discomfort he is in. Are there more good days or bad days (or hours or moments)? If you are able to put aside your fear of losing him and really *look,* you can often see when this time has arrived.

- Another guidepost that can help you is to ask yourself whether he still enjoys the things he always did. Is he still excited when you come home? Does he still look forward to meals or walks? Is he interactive, or does he now hide or sit separately from the family?

When pets lose their enjoyment of what they once loved, this can be a sign it may be time to let go. Many pets who are not feeling well, particularly cats, will find a spot away from everything and stay there by themselves most of the time.

● Keep in mind that there is no perfect moment, and that you will *never* feel ready to say good-bye. You are not ever going to feel okay about the thought of losing your pet. Sometimes it helps if you put yourself in the position of advising a friend: If this was my friend's pet, what would I advise? Or ask yourself: Several years ago, before I was in this position, what would I have thought would be the correct thing to do right now?

● If your pet is suffering from advanced age or terminal illness, remember that it is likely going to get worse. One purpose of euthanasia is to prevent future suffering.

Of course, this applies only to pets for whom there are no viable treatment options. It can be much more difficult to decide what to do when there are potential medical options for your pet, but you are not sure whether it would be fair to pursue further treatment. This situation is harder for me to counsel you on, since it is so individual, and your own veterinarian can offer more personal guidance for your pet's particular situation.

It may add to your peace of mind if you and your pet see the appropriate specialist for your pet's condition for a consultation. A specialist may be able to suggest helpful treatment options or even offer an alternative diagnosis. Even if he can't, you may feel more comfortable making decisions knowing you have explored every avenue for your pet.

At times, my clients have shared with me that they feel it is time to let go but can't bear the thought that they are "killing" their pets by having them euthanized. There is a very important fact for pet owners to recognize: *You* are not responsible for your pet's death. It is your pet's age or illness that is taking her away, and you can't change that; you are merely keeping some measure of control by at least being able to choose the time, place, and manner of her passing. If you are going to lose your pet to whatever ails her, at least you can spare her the suffering that would likely arise if you didn't step in. Don't give yourself more responsibility than you should actually bear.

What choices will I have to make?

There are several decisions you will have to make when it's time to say good-bye. Believe it or not, thinking these questions over beforehand and having some kind of plan will make it much less stressful when the actual moment arrives. There is nothing worse than being forced to make a host of difficult decisions when you are overwhelmed and heartbroken at having just lost your pet. By considering your options in advance, you allow yourself to focus completely on your pet when saying farewell. You are not betraying your pet or being morbid by thinking things through or discussing them with the rest of the family ahead of time.

Do you want the euthanasia to be performed at your veterinarian's office or at home? Most pets are euthanized at their veterinarian's office. Often the pets and their owners have a long history with the veterinarian, and this seems the most safe and comfortable option. Certainly if you know and trust a particular veterinarian, it can be a wise course to stick with this doctor. Additionally, having the procedure done at the office usually allows owners to leave afterward without having to deal with their pet's remains on their own, which can be upsetting and awkward.

However, some pet owners choose to have their pet euthanized in the home. You may already have been using a veterinarian who makes house calls, or your regular veterinarian may be willing to come by the house. If not, and you choose to use a house-call veterinarian who has never seen your pet, it's a good idea to have a detailed conversation over the phone when setting up the visit. For example, you will want to be sure that you are comfortable with the veterinarian's bedside manner, and to find out whether the veterinarian will be bringing an assistant or if you will need to take part in the process. You will also want to discuss what will happen afterward: Will you be responsible for taking care of your pet's remains, or will the house-call veterinarian be able to take your pet and make arrangements?

If you do want to have your pet euthanized at home when the time comes, it is best to figure out which doctor you will be using and have this type of conversation well in advance. If you get everything organized and then your pet rallies for several more days or weeks, you've lost nothing, but the last thing you need is to wait until your pet is in a crisis and then to be scrambling to make arrangements. Euthanasia of pets in the home can certainly be a wonderful option; I have assisted many of my clients in this way, and the experience has always been warm and positive. Advance planning, however, is key for things to go smoothly.

Do you want to be present at the actual euthanasia? Some people have no doubt that their place is right by their pet's side. Others know that this will be too much for them, and would prefer to say their good-byes beforehand. Various family members may feel differently from each other. I have often had one person in a couple choose to stay with the pet, while the other waits or takes a walk outside.

How would you like to handle your pet's remains? There are people who know exactly what they want to do after their pet is gone, but for others this can be a very difficult decision. Depending on where you live, you have various options available. In most areas, pets can be cremated by a pet cemetery or even by the veterinary practice itself. If you do choose to have your pet cremated, you will also have to decide whether you want to have your pet's ashes returned to you. Some people don't find the physical remains important, and have no desire to receive their pet's ashes. Others choose to keep the ashes in an urn or other commemorative container, or to bury or scatter the ashes in a favorite spot.

In some locations, there are pet cemeteries where owners can buy plots, just as for humans. Naturally, this can be quite costly. If you choose to bury your pet at home, be aware that there may be local regulations regarding pet burial. For a listing of pet cemeteries for cremation or burial in your area, you can go to www.pet-loss.net, or to the International Association of Pet Cemeteries and Crematories' website at www.iaopc.com and click on the list of members.

Personally, my choice in this matter has varied depending on the time of my life or my feelings at that moment. My dog Fritzie's ashes sit here by the desk in a small pottery container glazed with slightly ghostly dogs running through a misty field. Our two cats, who went within the space of a few months recently after sharing my life for almost eighteen years, are buried at my in-laws' house in the country, in a little plot that's so elaborately planted—even graced with a stone statue of a cat—that we have joked about future archaeologists who stumble across it and compare our society to the cat worshipers of ancient Egypt.

Would you like a postmortem exam to be performed? There are some instances in which pet owners may desire that a postmortem exam be performed on their animal. For example, the pet may have suffered from a mysterious illness, or may have had an infectious disease that could affect other pets in the household. In other cases, the veterinarian may suggest a postmortem be done, perhaps to learn more about the disease in the hope of helping future patients with a similar condition. Of course, it is always up to the pet owner whether to allow this, and a postmortem may not be performed without the client's permission.

If for whatever reason you would like a postmortem to be done, this is something you need to discuss in advance with the doctor if possible. Not all veterinarians are comfortable doing the procedure, and many will not perform it on another doctor's patient. Most veterinary schools offer this service; if there is a veterinary school within a reasonable distance, this is an option. Be aware that there is generally a charge for this, and be sure to get an estimate. It is also helpful to let the veterinarian who will be performing the postmortem know if you are planning to view your pet's body afterward.

How will my pet be euthanized? Are some ways better than others?

Pets are generally euthanized with a veterinary euthanasia solution that contains a powerful barbiturate. These products are designed to cause pets to lose awareness before they slip away. When the solution is given slowly through an intravenous catheter so that the animal gently loses consciousness, the process is quick and peaceful.

Most veterinarians give some type of sedative before administering the euthanasia solution. This relaxes the animal and allows a bit more of a transition period for the owner. I personally like to use a drug called propofol. This is a modern liquid anesthetic given intravenously that causes an animal to fall asleep very smoothly and peacefully with no sensation of dizziness or alarm. Once the animal is deeply unconscious from the propofol, I then administer the euthanasia solution. If I know that a particular animal is likely to object to the intravenous catheter, I may first give an injection under the skin of an opioid drug, such as one called butorphanol. (Opioids are sedating painkillers similar to codeine.) After five or ten minutes, the pet will generally be sleepy and calm enough for an IV catheter to be placed without stress to the animal.

It is my preference to avoid if possible the use of a drug called ketamine. This drug, which is similar to PCP (also known as angel dust), causes hallucinations, which I worry may be an alarming experience for the animal. In fact, I generally try to minimize the use of ketamine in my practice for this reason, among others.

Will anything scary happen when my pet is euthanized?

When performed properly, pet euthanasia is remarkably peaceful. Most clients who experience it for the first time are surprised by how smoothly it goes. If only we could all drift off unknowingly without pain or fear, attended by those we love most.

I do inform my clients of a few things it's good for them to be aware of in advance. Some are surprised that their pets' eyes do not close once the pet has slipped away; this is natural, but if desired, the veterinarian or nurse can close the animal's eyes. Due to muscle relaxation there may be a little puddle of urine; this is also perfectly normal and no cause for alarm. Rarely, a tiny muscle may twitch for a moment.

If you decide to spend a few minutes alone with your pet after he is gone, to say good-bye, don't be afraid to touch his fur or stroke him one last time. One of the things we all miss the most about pets we have lost is our physical contact with them.

AFTER YOUR PET IS GONE

Although many people experience similar feelings after the death of a pet (sometimes referred to as the stages of grief), the loss affects each of us a bit differently depending on the situation and our emotional makeup. A caring veterinarian can do much to ease a pet owner's pain: by open and supportive communication throughout the pet's illness, by ensuring if possible that the owner's last moments with the pet are as tranquil as possible, and by simply being there with warmth and understanding.

The empathy of the veterinarian for what the owner is going through is of particular importance since a grieving pet owner may not receive the type of support that is usually given to someone who has lost a human family member. Our society has mechanisms to help us deal with bereavement, including an outpouring of sympathy, an expectation that the bereaved person may be temporarily incapacitated, and ceremonial closure such as funerals, wakes, and memorial services. A person who has lost a pet is often expected to continue to work at their job and go on with their life as though nothing has happened. People do not generally send flower arrangements or drop by with casseroles.

Happily, this situation seems to be evolving. More and more clients tell me of the understanding of their friends and coworkers, who have often experienced a similar loss. People are eager to share their own stories, and society in general is increasingly accepting of the deep grief that many bereaved pet owners feel. After I lost my amazing cat Oshie to a brain tumor, I received a plethora of cards, phone calls, and flowers. Although these expressions of caring could not bring Oshie back to me, just knowing how many admirers he had won during his lifetime (he was a very social cat!) and that my friends understood what I was going through made all the difference to me.

If you are having trouble dealing with the loss of your pet, or feel that you need more support, there are quite a few resources available to help you. It is important that you reach out for help if you need it; many others have experienced the same feelings you are having, and communicating your emotions is an essential part of the healing process. A good website to help you find a grief counselor or pet-loss support group in your area and also for general information regarding the loss of a pet can be found at www.pet-loss.net. I have also provided a list below of the pet-loss support hotlines in various states around the country. You can turn to these resources not only after the loss of your pet, but also during a pet's illness or infirmity if you are feeling overwhelmed or need help making decisions.

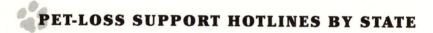 PET-LOSS SUPPORT HOTLINES BY STATE

Arizona

- Pet Grief Support Service, Phoenix: (602) 995-5885

California

- University of California–Davis Veterinary School: (800) 565-1526

Colorado

- Colorado State University Argus Institute: (970) 297-1242

Florida

- University of Florida Veterinary School: (352) 392-2235, then dial 1, then 4080

Illinois

- Chicago Veterinary Medical Association: (630) 325-1600
- University of Illinois College of Veterinary Medicine: (877) 394-CARE (2273)

Iowa

- Iowa State University College of Veterinary Medicine: (888) ISU-PLSH (478-7574)

Massachusetts

- Tufts University School of Veterinary Medicine: (508) 839-7966

Michigan

- Michigan State University Veterinary School: (517) 432-2696

New York

- Cornell University College of Veterinary Medicine: (607) 253-3932

Ohio

- Ohio State University School of Veterinary Medicine: (614) 292-1823

Virginia

- Virginia-Maryland Regional College of Veterinary Medicine: (540) 231-8038

Washington

- Washington State University College of Veterinary Medicine: (509) 335-5704

PET LOSS AND
EUTHANASIA: WORKSHEET

You can use this worksheet to get your thoughts and plans organized so that your mind will be clear when it is time to say good-bye.

- Do I feel comfortable that I have explored all my pet's medical options to my satisfaction? Have I seen my veterinarian about my pet's condition, or consulted with a specialist if indicated?

- Do I want my pet euthanized at my veterinarian's office or at home? If it will be at home, does my veterinarian perform this service? If not, have I located another veterinarian with whom I am comfortable?

- Do I want a postmortem exam to be performed on my pet? If so, have I made the proper arrangements? If I would like to view my pet after the postmortem, have I made the veterinarian aware of this?

- Do I want to remain with my pet when she is euthanized? How do the other members of my family feel?

- Do I want the veterinarian to clip a lock of my pet's hair to have as a keepsake?

- What do I want to do with my pet's remains?

- If I have my pet cremated, do I want the cremation to be performed individually and to have her ashes returned to me? Or am I comfortable with group cremation and do not want her ashes returned?

- If I choose to bury my pet, where will she be buried? Will it be at home or at a pet cemetery? If I have her buried at home, do I want to obtain some sort of box or casket in advance?

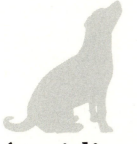

Avoiding Pet Debt:

Tips on Managing Health Care Costs

When you bring home a new pet, there is so much to look forward to: fun with a roly-poly puppy, laughter at the antics of a kitten, long walks with a dog, cozy snuggles with a cat. Naturally, your focus isn't on worries about health care. You probably plan on seeing the veterinarian for checkups and vaccinations periodically; having your pet spayed or neutered if that hasn't already been done; and investing in flea, tick, and heartworm preventives. Beyond that, you don't expect to be spending much time at the animal hospital. You realize that in the distant future, as your pet becomes elderly, some kind of medical care will likely become necessary, but hopefully that time is far off.

It's true that there are pets who sail through life without any problems well into their old age. I love it when someone brings in a fifteen-year-old dog or a nineteen-year-old cat who has gotten a bit creaky and is in for a tune-up but hasn't had any real health issues. In fact, I give strict orders to each new pet who joins my household that this is what I expect from them.

But of course the reality is that most pets will sooner or later have some type of health problem requiring veterinary attention. It might be something relatively minor, like an upset stomach from a foray into the kitchen trash. It could be something more involved, such as a pet who needs emergency surgery to remove a swallowed toy or to fix a broken leg. And unfortunately, a serious issue that requires more long-term care may arise in some pets, such as diabetes, asthma, or a problem in one of the organs.

Most of us try to plan ahead financially—for child care, education, retirement, and so on. It's important to plan in this same fashion for your pet's health care. When a pet needs help, especially in a crisis, the last thing you want while concerned about your pet's condition is to also have the stress of figuring out how to afford the medical care required. There are various ways to go about preparing for the costs of veterinary care, including pet health insurance, dedicated saving accounts, and credit programs. In this chapter, I'll talk about some of your options, and also about how you can greatly decrease the chance of health problems arising in the first place.

PREVENTIVE CARE

"An ounce of prevention is worth a pound of cure"—isn't it funny how all those old sayings really are true? When you think about the various types of preventive care that veterinarians recommend, such as vaccinations, deworming, and products that guard against fleas, ticks, and heartworms, you may not consider the financial savings they can bring. Not only does good preventive care help to protect the health of your pet, but it also helps to protect the health of your wallet! The same is true of having your pet spayed or neutered, which is one of the best health care investments you can make for your dog or cat.

Even the most conscientious pet owner may not realize that the health benefits of thorough preventive care are accompanied by financial benefits as well. People sometimes suspect that veterinarians are trying to make money by pushing vaccines and other services. Unfortunately, this impression can lead to avoidance of regular veterinary care, with potentially quite costly consequences, and often to the pet's ultimate detriment. If you truly feel that the veterinary practice you're using would make recommendations that are financially motivated, it's time to talk this through with your pet's doctor, or go elsewhere. Find a veterinarian you trust, who will work with you to create a personalized health care regimen for your pet.

Let's talk about how various types of preventive care can help minimize your veterinary bills while protecting your pet's health.

Vaccinations

The most important concerns regarding infectious diseases of dogs and cats are the suffering that a sick pet will experience, and the possibility that the animal may not survive the illness. These are the primary reasons to be sure your pet is well vaccinated. However, another very good reason to have your pet vaccinated is the fact that the cost of vaccination is far lower than that of treating the illnesses that vaccines can prevent. In the chapter on vaccines, I presented a variety of illnesses of dogs and cats against which vaccination is possible. Now let's talk about the costs involved in treating an animal who is stricken by one of these infections.

For example, both dogs and cats can be infected by parvoviruses, which are extremely contagious organisms that live for long periods in the environment. These viruses can persist in locations where an infected animal has been present, such as a sidewalk, park, or yard. The viruses can be carried into your home on shoes or other objects. As I discussed in chapter 3, proper vaccination generally provides excellent immunity against parvoviral infection.

When an animal is infected by a parvovirus, the illness that develops is life threatening. Dogs with canine parvovirus and cats with feline panleukopenia (feline distemper caused by a parvovirus) develop severe vomiting and diarrhea that usually persist for a number of days. Their white blood cell count drops very low due to bone marrow damage by the virus, and this means that their immune system cannot function effectively. Treatment of parvoviral illness requires hospitalization, intravenous fluids, intravenous antibiotics, medications to counteract vomiting, and often other therapy as well. Some animals do not survive the infection, especially those who do not receive aggressive intensive care. The current cost of effectively treating a dog or cat who has been sickened by a parvovirus is often several thousand dollars.

It can be quite costly to treat any of the infectious diseases that may occur in unvaccinated animals. Canine adenovirus, feline herpesvirus, and feline calicivirus, as well as *Bordetella* bacteria in both dogs and cats, can all cause very serious respiratory infections, including pneumonia. Treatment often requires hospitalization, with intravenous fluids and antibiotics, and oxygen therapy in some cases. Leptospirosis infection in dogs results in life-threatening kidney and liver damage that necessitates hospitalization and aggressive therapy as well. Canine distemper can cause intestinal, respiratory, and neurological symptoms in dogs who are infected, and is unfortunately often fatal even with treatment.

As discussed in chapter 3, the vaccines that have been designated as core and are recommended for all pets generally protect against infectious diseases that are very common. It is difficult to protect even an indoor pet against these infections without vaccination, since we may inadvertently bring the organisms into our homes as we come and go. I also remind clients who ask me why indoor pets should be vaccinated that if an animal should ever become ill and require hospitalization—for example, a cat who swallows a piece of string and needs intestinal surgery, or a dog who develops a bladder stone that must be removed—the unvaccinated animal will be at high risk in the veterinary facility, where there are many sick animals in close proximity. Since these kinds of events are unpredictable, and most animals wind up in the veterinary hospital for one reason or another at some point, it is wise to ensure that all pets are fully immunized.

It is a heartbreaking situation when a family cannot afford treatment for a beloved pet who develops a serious infectious disease that could have been prevented by vaccination. Veterinarians encounter this dilemma all too frequently. Most people can afford vaccinations for their pets, but for some it is difficult to handle the cost of a bout of infectious illness. Vaccines are an excellent investment in preventing this predicament.

Spay and Neuter Procedures

Many people know about the tragic issue of pet overpopulation and that our shelters are full of animals hoping for a home. Although this is certainly an excellent reason to have your pet spayed or neutered, you may not be aware of the numerous health benefits of these procedures, and how much money they can save you in the long run.

Spaying a female pet: There are a variety of diseases that can be prevented by having your female pet spayed (the proper term for spaying is ovariohysterectomy: removal of the uterus and ovaries). The two most commonly seen examples are pyometra and mammary gland tumors. Pyometra is a common condition in which the uterus becomes infected and fills with pus. Animals with pyometra become extremely ill and require

Quick Quiz

The best reason to have your female pet spayed is:

A. The veterinarian needs money to send her kids to college.

B. You can't get any sleep because your cat is in heat and she cries constantly.

C. All the male dogs in the neighborhood are using your lawn as a urinal because your female dog is in heat.

D. Spaying your pet greatly decreases the risk of breast cancer in dogs and cats.

Answer: D. Dogs who are not spayed are two thousand times more likely to develop breast cancer than dogs spayed before their first heat cycle. Female cats who are not spayed have 91 percent more risk of developing breast cancer than a cat spayed before six months of age.

emergency surgery to remove the infected uterus. In some cases, the uterus may rupture before surgery can be performed, causing a dangerous condition called peritonitis, similar to what occurs in humans with a ruptured appendix.

Pyometra occurs frequently in unspayed dogs and cats. For example, one study found that about a quarter of unspayed female dogs develop pyometra by the time they reach ten years of age! Unfortunately, many animals with pyometra do not show obvious signs until they are gravely ill. Thus, they must undergo anesthesia and surgery when they are in critical condition and more likely to suffer complications. The costs of preoperative stabilization, surgery, anesthesia, and postoperative care can mount up to well over a thousand dollars—or even twice that much. Some dogs and cats with pyometra also suffer kidney damage due to circulating bacterial toxins and dehydration, necessitating an even longer hospital stay.

Since animals with pyometra require immediate surgical removal of the uterus, it makes much more sense to have your pet spayed as an elective procedure when she's healthy, the procedure and recovery will be brief, and costs will be a fraction of that associated with the same operation performed once pyometra has developed. There are many low-cost options for having pets spayed, but these programs can't help pets who are already ill.

Mammary gland tumors (breast cancer) are also very common in unspayed dogs and cats. Mammary gland tumors are the most common kind of cancer in female dogs and the third most common type of cancer in female cats. In studies on beagles, for example, 63 to 71 percent of unspayed females developed mammary gland tumors at some point. Luckily, spaying is extremely helpful in protecting dogs and cats from breast cancer. The statistics are quite dramatic and indicate that not only is it prudent to have dogs and cats spayed in order to prevent this cancer, but it is also advisable that the procedure be performed at a young age, if possible, before the animal has had a chance to go into her first heat (reproductive) cycle.

Compared with a dog who is not spayed, a dog who is spayed before her first heat occurs has 0.05 percent as much chance of developing breast cancer. In other words, an unspayed female is two thousand times more likely to develop mammary gland tumors than one who is spayed before she goes into heat! A dog who is spayed after one heat cycle has only 8 percent as much chance of developing breast cancer as an unspayed female, and a dog spayed after two heat cycles has 26 percent as much chance of developing breast cancer—about one-quarter the likelihood of an unspayed dog.

In cats, spaying is also protective against mammary gland tumors. A recent study demonstrated that cats spayed by six months of age have 91 percent less risk of developing breast cancer than unspayed cats, and cats spayed by one year of age have 86 percent less risk compared with those who are not spayed. Since feline mammary tumors tend to be highly malignant, it is well worth ensuring that your cat is spayed before she ever goes into heat, if possible. My own cat was sick with intestinal problems when the time came to have her spayed, and I was very worried that she would go into heat before she was well enough to have the procedure. Luckily, this did not happen, but I would have been devastated if it had, having seen the consequences all too often in feline patients with terminal breast cancer that has metastasized.

Prevention of breast cancer in dogs and cats through spaying is a worthwhile investment for both your pet's health and your finances. The cost of spaying a healthy animal is far less than that of surgery for mammary tumors, not to mention the associated costs such as blood work, X-rays to check for metastasis, the hospital stay, and possibly chemotherapy. Dogs and cats who develop mammary tumors often later develop tumors in additional mammary glands, and it is common for more than one surgery to be needed. Many pets require radical mastectomies, in which multiple glands are removed simultaneously.

Of course, beyond the cost factor, it is tragic for both the owner and pet when an animal is stricken by cancer that may have been avoided. Since breast cancer is often fatal in pets, and is so readily preventable, it is recommended that both dogs and cats be spayed before six months of age, in order to benefit from the highest level of protection. Spaying dogs and cats also prevents cancer of the uterus or ovaries.

Other advantages include a reduced risk of diabetes in female dogs and avoidance of unplanned pregnancies with the associated medical costs, which may include cesarean section in some animals. Pregnant dogs and cats may experience dystocia, the term for a difficult delivery, and medical bills can be extensive, particularly when surgery is required. Of course, not only will the pregnant female require care, but the resultant puppies and kittens will also need vaccinations, deworming, and so on. Since even indoor animals can slip out and become pregnant, the simplest and most cost-saving solution is to prevent this possibility by having your pet spayed before her heat cycles begin.

Neutering a male pet: Neutering a male pet (generally performed by surgical removal of the testicles, although an injection is available that can be used instead in some cases) can also help to prevent disease and to keep costs down. There are a variety of ways in which neutering will protect your pet as well as pay off financially.

In male dogs who are not neutered, diseases of the prostate gland are common at middle age and beyond. The gland becomes progressively enlarged due to hormonal stimulation, a condition known as benign prostatic hyperplasia (BPH). As BPH advances with time, it often leads to bacterial prostatic infections (prostatitis) and even cysts and abscesses of the prostate, which can necessitate emergency surgery if severe. The enlarged gland can also cause difficulty with defecation. Of course, surgical neutering prevents testicular cancer as well as protecting against most prostatic disease. Unfortunately, neutering does not decrease the likelihood of canine prostatic cancer.

Male dogs and cats who are not neutered are also in other types of danger. Because of strong mating drive, they will often work very hard to escape from the house or yard, and are more apt to roam far from home. Because of this, unneutered males are at higher risk of being hit by cars or suffering other accidents on their travels. They are more likely to become lost, and prone to fighting with other males. Fighting in turn leads to bite wounds, which generally require veterinary care involving antibiotics and possibly surgery. In male cats, the tendency to fight can also result in infection with feline immunodeficiency virus (FIV), analogous to HIV. All of these issues can lead to veterinary bills that might have been avoided, not to mention serious health consequences for the pets themselves.

Neutering of male pets can also decrease the likelihood of behavioral issues that can be frustrating and costly. Male tomcats often mark their territory by urine spraying, and beyond the fact that this results in quite a malodorous home, it can become fairly expensive as you find yourself replacing shoes, rugs, and other objects that have been chosen for marking activity! Male dogs who are neutered are also less likely to display marking behavior. Neutering male dogs has also been shown to decrease the probability of aggression toward humans or other dogs, as well as undesirable habits such as mounting, although it does not eliminate the possibility of these behaviors.

Heartworm Prevention

Heartworm disease is a life-threatening parasitic infestation that affects both dogs and cats. Heartworm infection is passed from animal to animal through mosquito bites and results in the growth of worms in the heart and other areas of the body, such as blood vessels. This can result in heart damage and failure, as well as lung disease and other health complications. Although decades ago, heartworm infection in pets occurred only in certain geographic areas, the disease has now spread across the United States.

Studies have indicated that the majority of dogs in the United States are not on heartworm preventive medication, although it is difficult to determine precise percentages. Considering that heartworm disease is life threatening to pets, and that monthly preventives are quite inexpensive and very effective, this is unfortunate. Pets of all lifestyles are at risk of infection; I have diagnosed toy-breed dogs who rarely leave their urban apartments with heartworm disease, much to the surprise of their owners.

Many pet owners do not realize that cats can also be infected with heartworms. Although infection is more common in cats who go outside, it can also occur in those who live entirely indoors. Oral and topical monthly heartworm preventives are available for both dogs and cats, some of which also provide protection against intestinal parasites. Your veterinarian can advise you on the best product and regimen for your pet.

Flea and Tick Control

Depending on where you live and your pet's lifestyle, your veterinarian may recommend that you use a monthly flea and/or tick preventive for your pet. In some areas of the country, especially those where it is warm year-round, pets may need flea and tick control all year. Other areas only require use of these preventives during certain seasons. Prescription products currently available are quite effective at preventing flea infestation, and often protect pets against tick bites as well.

Many of these products now come in the form of topical solutions that are placed on a small area of the animal's skin monthly, and are very easy to use. It's important for you to speak with your veterinarian about which preventive is best for your particular pet, since there is a confusing array of products on the market, with differing purposes and activities. Parasite control offered by a particular product may be against fleas, ticks, or both fleas and ticks, and even against heartworm disease and other internal parasites as well.

How can these products help you to keep your veterinary health care costs down? Similar to what I discussed regarding vaccination, it is generally more costly to treat the conditions that occur as a result of flea or tick infestation than to prevent such infestation in the first place. Beyond the benefits to your pet in terms of both health and comfort (imagine how it would feel to have thousands of fleas biting you and crawling on your skin twenty-four hours a day!), protecting your pet from fleas and ticks can also protect you from the medical costs of dealing with the havoc these little pests can wreak.

Fleas: Flea infestation on a dog or cat can have consequences that range from relatively mild to quite severe. The most common problems arising from fleas affect the animal's skin. Effects on the skin include itchiness, widespread dermatitis (inflammation of the skin), secondary bacterial infections, flea allergies, and hot spots (open, infected sores that cause the pet extreme discomfort). Cats with fleas can develop a condition called miliary dermatitis, a bumpy rash over the skin surface, or another called eosinophilic granuloma complex, a serious inflammatory disease that can affect the skin, lips, and mouth.

Animals with fleas can also become anemic due to blood loss (fleas survive on blood from the animals they infest). Severe flea anemia requires treatment with blood transfusions, and can be fatal if not discovered and treated promptly. This is particularly true in kittens and puppies, but can also occur in adult animals who are heavily infested. Fleas can also transmit a variety of infectious diseases in dogs and cats, such as *Bartonella* (a bacterial infection) and hemoplasmas (blood parasites). Treatment of health conditions caused by fleas, from skin issues to anemia to infectious diseases, is likely to be far more costly than appropriate flea prevention would have been.

Ticks: Depending on geographic location and your pet's lifestyle, ticks can be a major health concern, since multiple diseases of dogs and cats are spread by ticks. If you live in an area where ticks are found, it is advisable to use tick prevention for your pet, in addition to performing manual tick checks of the animal's body. You can ask your veterinarian about the prevalence of ticks in your area and which product is recommended for your pet. During seasons and activities when your pet is at risk, it's a good idea to also get into the habit of thoroughly examining him each day for the presence of ticks. It takes time for diseases to be transmitted once a tick has attached to the skin, so prompt removal can help to prevent tick-borne infections from occurring.

Diseases that are spread to pets by ticks of various types include:

- Lyme disease—a bacterial infection that can cause arthritis in dogs, as well as heart, kidney, and neurological damage.

- Rocky Mountain spotted fever—a bacterial infection of dogs causing inflammation of blood vessels, bleeding, bruising, and swelling of the limbs.

- Ehrlichiosis—a bacterial infection of dogs causing enlarged lymph nodes, decreased cell counts, and bleeding. Although not as commonly seen in North America, feline ehrlichiosis can also occur.

- Bartonellosis—a bacterial infection that affects cats and dogs, and can also be transmitted to humans.

- Babesiosis—an infection with blood parasites that causes anemia in dogs.

- Hepatozoonosis—an infection of dogs by a microscopic parasite causing fever, muscle pain, and kidney damage. Dogs become infected by eating an infected tick rather than through a tick bite.

This parasite can also infect cats, although less is known about the disease in felines.

- Cytauxzoonosis—a blood parasite infection of cats causing fever, difficulty breathing, jaundice, and shock.

- *Mycoplasma haemofelis*—a blood parasite causing anemia in cats.

- Tick paralysis—not an infection, but rather a temporary paralysis of dogs caused by a neurological toxin released by ticks.

As you can see by the wide array of diseases caused by ticks, it is a worthwhile investment in your pet's health to prevent exposure to these parasites. Some tick-borne infections are grave and often fatal, such as cytauxzoonosis in cats, and all of these diseases are very serious. You should discuss with your veterinarian which diseases occur in your area, and make a plan to protect your pet from infection.

Secondhand Cigarette Smoke

By now, hopefully, we are all aware of the risks posed by cigarette smoking, to both the smoker and those exposed to secondhand smoke. However, I have found that many pet owners are not aware of the danger they are putting their pets in by smoking in the home. An owner of a pet with cancer will often ask me what could have caused the disease, when the animal's fur smells strongly of cigarette smoke. It is very difficult to tell people that their habit may have harmed their beloved pet.

For those who choose to smoke, this is a conscious choice. For pets in

---

Quick Quiz

Which of the following are good reasons not to smoke if you have pets?

A. Secondhand smoke can cause serious lung diseases in pets, such as asthma and bronchitis.

B. Secondhand smoke increases the risk of pet cancers, such as oral and nasal cancer, lymphoma, and lung cancer.

C. When you smoke in the house, your pet can't escape or ask you to stop.

D. All of the above.

Answer: D. All of the answers are true.

the home with a smoker, there is no choice. And unlike other members of the household who are out at work or other activities much of the time, many pets spend almost all of their time in the house and are thus potentially exposed to even higher levels of toxins than the humans in the home. Additionally, due to self-grooming behavior, pets are likely to ingest toxic particles from cigarette smoke as well as inhaling them. This factor is believed to be one reason that cats living with people who smoke have higher rates of oral cancer; carcinogens on the fur are deposited in the mouth when cats lick themselves.

Smoking not only increases the risk of cancer in pets, but can also lead to chronic lung diseases such as asthma and bronchitis. Pets with these conditions need medication and periodic X-rays; they frequently end up at the veterinary emergency clinic in a respiratory crisis. If your own health is not enough reason to quit smoking, do it for your pet (and your bank account). Otherwise, at least protect your pet by smoking outside, just as you do at work to protect your coworkers.

Dental Care

Dental disease is very common in pets and affects virtually every pet sooner or later. Some animals develop dental disease surprisingly early, often due to a genetic predisposition. For example, small dogs and brachycephalic (flat-faced) breeds of dogs and cats are more prone to problems with their teeth, and often at a younger age than other pets. If you think about it, this makes sense: A flat-faced animal must squeeze the same number of teeth into a much shorter jaw than usual, and this crowding causes abnormal placement of the teeth and various problems with oral health.

Dental conditions such as plaque, gingivitis, and periodontitis can cause oral problems ranging from halitosis (bad breath) or discomfort (which can lead to a decreased appetite or difficulty eating) to very serious infections. However, the chronic inflammation taking place in pets with gingivitis and periodontitis can affect the animal's overall health as well, causing damage over time to organs such as the kidneys. Someone whose pet develops kidney failure may not realize that long-term dental disease could be the culprit. Additionally, studies into the causes of aging in humans and animals have demonstrated that this type of chronic inflammation is one of the major contributors to the process.

The best kind of dental care is preventive. Rather than waiting for a

Check Out Receipt

Saline District Library
734-429-5450
http://salinelibrary.org

Tuesday, July 11, 2017 1:57:14 PM

Title: The nature of animal healing : the
path to your pet's health, happiness, and
longevity
Call no.: 636.089 Gol
Due: 08/08/2017

Title: Vet confidential : an insider's gui
de to keeping your pet healthy and safe
Call no.: 636.089 Mur
Due: 08/08/2017

Total items: 2

****
You can now pay your library fines
online at http://salinelibrary.org

critical problem to develop, such as an abscessed tooth, it is best to be proactive. When you get a new pet, try to establish a regimen of daily dental care if possible (be careful until you are sure your pet will be cooperative!). The younger your pet when you start this, the better chance you have of success. The teeth can be cleaned in just a few moments each day. Dental care products, such as pet toothbrushes and flavored pastes, are available through your veterinarian. A soft brush or pad that fits onto your fingertip often works well. Pastes, gels, and other products may be helpful if your pet does not object to them, but it is the physical cleaning you perform that is most important.

TIP Never use human toothpaste on your pet. Products intended for humans can be harmful if swallowed, and most pets hate the taste and the foaming that occurs.

When beginning a dental hygiene program, it's best to slowly accustom your pet to the process over a number of days. First, carefully practice touching her face and gently lifting her lips. Once she allows this, try rubbing your finger along her teeth for a moment, always using appropriate caution for your own safety. It's not necessary to hold your pet's mouth open; simply slide your finger along the outside surface of the teeth. After a few days of this, show your pet the toothbrush and allow her to sniff it, or let her taste the product and tell you if she likes it. Rub a little of the product on her gums with your finger. Then gradually begin to introduce whichever cleaning tool you've chosen into her mouth, at first only for a moment. As she becomes accustomed to the ritual, you can begin to clean the teeth more completely. After each session, reward your pet with praise or a treat.

Although a vigilant home regimen will decrease the frequency with which professional dental care is needed, your pet will still benefit from periodic cleanings at a veterinarian's office (just as we need regular dental cleanings even though we brush our teeth). Many pet owners put off professional dental care until absolutely necessary. Rather than scheduling routine cleanings, they wait until a major problem forces the issue. There are serious drawbacks to this tactic.

For one thing, the likelihood of the procedure being much more involved skyrockets: Instead of straightforward cleaning and polishing, the pet may need multiple extractions of teeth that are beyond hope, for example. Not only does this increase the pet's discomfort and the chance of complications, but it also becomes far more expensive. Additionally, by delaying professional dental care, the risk of overall health consequences secondary to chronic periodontal disease is magnified.

Pet owners often wonder why dental cleanings require anesthesia in pets. They may have known veterinarians who will scrape the teeth of a conscious animal, and wonder if another doctor's insistence on anesthesia is misplaced or even financially motivated. The truth is that proper dental cleaning in pets requires anesthesia; simply scraping the teeth actually does more harm than good. It is essential to clean and probe beneath the gum line, which cannot be done to a pet who is awake; and mechanical polishing after cleaning is crucial, since this decreases the recurrence of plaque and gingivitis. Scraping without polishing roughens the surface of the teeth and actually increases the number of bacteria that live there.

The best strategy for preventing serious dental disease in your pet, with the resultant costs and health consequences, is to clean the teeth daily at home (or as often as your schedule allows), and to assess the need for professional dental care at each visit to your veterinarian. The necessary frequency will depend on your pet's breed, size, diet, and other factors, and your veterinarian can tell you when it's time for a cleaning. Some pets, particularly those with serious dental or oral disease, will also benefit from a visit to a board-certified veterinary dental specialist (the location of one in your area can be found at www.avdc.org).

It's not a coincidence that proper preventive care, using all the approaches I have discussed above, is the best way to protect both your pet *and* your finances. Just as in most areas of life, from auto and home maintenance to personal relationships, regular upkeep is key to preventing problems from developing. Waiting for a crisis to arise before taking action is always more costly (and hazardous) in the long run. There's another old saying that any veterinarian can tell you is true: "A stitch in time saves nine." Vaccinations, spaying and neutering, heartworm prevention, good dental care . . . these are all "stitches in time" that may save you a lot more than nine (dollars, that is!).

FINANCIAL STRATEGIES

For any concerned pet owner, veterinary bills are a fact of life. Whether costs are for routine preventive care and checkups, or for a minor or major illness, we must be prepared. Part of being responsible pet owners is developing strategies to manage health care expenses, and doing what we can to avoid situations in which we are unable to provide a pet with needed care because of monetary restrictions. Of course, each pet owner has a unique financial situation and must work within the parameters that are possible given that reality. Pet health care decisions must be made within your own financial comfort zone. However, the predicament to avoid is one in which you find yourself suddenly faced with a veterinary bill you cannot afford, or wishing you could provide care that is beyond your reach but might have been possible with advance planning.

There are several possibilities for providing yourself and your pet with a financial safety net. These include pet insurance, credit programs, and dedicated bank accounts. Which is best for you depends on a variety of factors. The most important thing is to be honest with yourself. Are you the organized type with willpower galore? If so, perhaps committing to putting an allotted monthly amount into a savings account at your own bank will work for you. In this way, you have an emergency fund for both yourself and your pet, and your money can accrue interest in the meantime. Or do you recognize that you are the type who needs a more structured plan that forces you to contribute periodically, such as a pet insurance program? Let's look at some of your options, and then you can decide what will work for you.

Health Insurance for Pets

Currently, a number of pet insurance companies offer policies for dogs and cats (and some for other animals as well). If you are considering obtaining health insurance for your pet, there are a variety of factors to weigh. You must select which company to use, and usually also choose from a menu of available plans that have varying costs and levels of coverage. You want to pick the company and policy that best fit your financial needs and that will allow you to provide your pet with the degree of care you desire.

When investigating pet insurance policies, be sure to read the fine print! You need to make sure you really understand what is covered and what isn't so that you can compare various companies and their different plans logically. Because it can be pretty hard to follow all the details, I like companies that have very clear and user-friendly websites, where it is easy to find all the information you need without having to dig around like Sherlock Holmes. So start out by taking a look at each company's website and deciding whether you can readily get the facts you require there. Make a short list of the ones you like, and then start comparing their policies based on the factors covered in this chapter as well as any others that are important to you.

You'll find that monthly premiums for pet insurance currently range from as low as ten dollars up to around ninety. The amount varies with the company and the coverage offered, as well as other variables discussed below. Your pet's age will be a factor, and some companies have differing premiums for dogs versus cats. The most limited policies only cover accidents; broader (and more expensive) policies offer a range of coverage that may only include illness or may help with preventive care as well. It is important to consider all of these variables and to fully understand the coverage being offered before you choose a plan for your pet, and to review your choice each year before renewing.

Coverage of preventive care: Some pet insurance policies offer coverage for preventive care, such as vaccinations, heartworm and flea prevention, dental care, and spay/neuter procedures; others do not. Although coverage for preventive care generally pays only a portion of the cost, if you are the type of pet owner who is good about keeping up with yearly checkups and other preventive measures (and you probably are if you are reading this book), you might want to consider a plan that will help to offset the cost. Of course, the other side of the coin is that purchasing a plan that helps to pay for preventive care may motivate you to obtain such care for your pet, which is a good thing.

If you are considering a plan that covers preventive care, be sure that the benefits you receive outweigh the higher premium you will likely be paying. This should be fairly easy to figure out with your veterinarian's help. By discussing what preventive care your pet will likely require during the period to be covered by the policy, and getting an estimate of the costs involved, you should be able to tell if the higher premium will be worth it. Since your pet's needs will change from year to year, be sure to review and update this information with your veterinarian each year before renewing.

Set benefit schedules: Some insurance companies use what is called a benefit schedule. This means that they only allow a certain amount of coverage per health condition. For example, a company may limit reimbursement for a dog with parvovirus infection to four to six hundred dollars, depending on the plan the owner has selected, or allow only two or three hundred dollars for chemotherapy. The set limits tend to vary with which plan you've chosen from that company's menu; plans with higher monthly premiums generally have more generous benefit schedules.

Other companies do not use benefit schedules; instead they cover a certain percentage of medical costs. For example, you may have a copay of 10 to 30 percent depending on the company and policy you select, and the insurance company will cover the remaining 90 to 70 percent of the veterinary bill, usually after an annual or per-incident deductible. Although this type of policy may not limit the amount that can be reimbursed for a certain condition, there is often an annual or per-incident maximum amount for coverage, and this will vary with which plan you choose. A plan with higher monthly premiums will generally have a higher annual maximum for coverage provided.

When choosing between plans with set benefit schedules versus those that pay a percentage of costs, you should consider the price of veterinary care in your area. If you live in an area where surgery and aftercare for a pet who has swallowed a toy is likely to cost two thousand dollars, you may not want to select a plan that allows only seven hundred for this situation, unless you can comfortably afford to pay the difference.

It may be worth speaking to your veterinary practice before selecting a plan, and getting cost estimates for a few common conditions to serve as guideposts. For example, you could ask your veterinary practice what it would approximately cost for intestinal surgery for a foreign body (swallowed object), or for inpatient treatment of a bout of gastroenteritis (upset stomach with vomiting and diarrhea). Be sure to ask them to give you an estimate of the total cost from start to finish, with everything involved.

Then compare these estimates with the benefit schedule for each condition set by the insurance company you are considering. If the benefit schedule covers a reasonable portion of your veterinarian's estimate for that situation, the plan may work for you. If it doesn't even come close, you may want to consider a plan that pays a straightforward percentage of the bill. Keep in mind that various plans offered by the same company (at differing monthly premiums) may offer a range of benefit schedules. You can use the estimates provided by your veterinary practice to see how your benefits from various policies with comparable monthly premiums would stack up.

Deductibles: Most pet insurance policies involve some sort of deductible. This may be an annual deductible, or the deductible may be per visit or per incident. Be sure to consider this when choosing a plan. For example, a plan with a lower monthly premium may appear to be more cost-effective, but if there is a per-visit deductible, it may not be the bargain it seems. Of course this will depend on how often your pet visits the veterinarian, but unfortunately this can be difficult to predict. If your pet is of a breed or age likely to require lots of ongoing health maintenance, you may want to choose a plan with an annual deductible rather than a per-visit deductible.

Annual and per-incident maximums: Some pet insurance companies set annual maximums for coverage provided. The annual maximum generally varies with the particular plan you select. Be sure to check the annual maximum of any policy you consider, and keep in mind your own philosophy regarding medical care for your pets. If you would be heartbroken if you could not provide your pet with the absolutely highest level of care for a serious illness, you need to be sure that your annual maximum is not overly restrictive.

However, higher annual maximums come at a price, and may not be as important for many young pets as for older ones. Any pet can suffer a major illness or accident, but the chance of a serious health issue requiring more costly care such as advanced diagnostics or prolonged hospitalization increases as your pet becomes older. Older pets are also more likely to need ongoing care that really adds up over a year.

Be careful about per-incident maximums. If this is a feature of a policy you are considering, be sure you understand exactly what this means. If your pet develops a skin condition one month, and then develops a skin condition again later in the year, will it be considered the same incident? This type of situation can be subject to interpretation, so annual maximums may be a safer bet. Additionally, since individual pets tend to suffer the same problems over and over (just as individual people have their own particular recurring health issues), you may never reach your annual maximum if your per-incident maximum limits coverage for similar or recurring conditions.

For example, my cat Siena is plagued by chronic intestinal problems. The first year I had her, she was frequently ill and ended up needing two intestinal surgeries. If I had had an insurance policy with a per-incident maximum that limited my reimbursement for her gastrointestinal issues, it wouldn't have mattered if my allowed annual maximum was a million dollars. I would have been stuck at the per-incident maximum, since my cat's problems all related to her tummy.

A similar concept would be a per-system maximum, in which there is limited coverage for problems occurring in the same bodily organ system. For the same reasons as for per-incident maximums, you should be cautious about this type of policy.

Coverage for chronic conditions: Some pets develop health issues that require long-term treatment. Examples include diabetes, asthma, arthritis, and kidney disease. Insurance companies differ in their coverage of these conditions. Some offer twelve-month policies, where coverage is for one year. At the end of that time period, conditions that arose during the year are now considered preexisting, and are no longer covered. Going back to the example of my cat Siena, the ongoing intestinal problems she has suffered from the time she was a kitten would not be covered after the first year with this type of policy. If you want to ensure that your pet will receive lifetime coverage for chronic health problems, you need to select a policy that provides this service.

The issue of coverage for chronic conditions becomes more and more important as your pet ages. Although a young animal may develop a persistent health issue, these conditions are much more common in middle-aged and older pets; many health problems of older pets do require long-term care, just as is the case in people. Of course, you must obtain this type of coverage if desired *before* your pet develops an issue, since most companies will not cover preexisting conditions. Keep this in mind as your pet approaches middle age.

Coverage for hereditary diseases and disorders: If you have a purebred cat or dog, this is a very important factor to consider when choosing a health insurance plan for your pet! Most breeds are prone to certain health problems, and some insurance companies do not cover such hereditary disorders. These disorders are common because the breeding of purebred animals involves the mating of related individuals, in order that animals of the breed all share certain characteristics. This practice increases the likelihood that genetic defects will occur. To understand why, we'll need to revisit your high school biology class and talk a little about genetics.

Genes are the basic units of heredity. A gene is a piece of DNA that contains information about a hereditary characteristic, such as eye color, hair color, height, or which diseases the individual is prone to develop. Each of us has thousands and thousands of genes, which we inherit from our parents. Genes are the code passed from parents to offspring that make us who we are, for better or worse.

I'm sure you remember dominant and recessive genes from biology class. In the illustration below, the gene for brown eyes is represented by big B and is dominant; the gene for blue eyes is represented by little b and is recessive. Each parent gives the offspring one of their two genes for eye color. If someone inherits two genes for brown eyes (BB), she will have brown eyes, and if another person inherits two genes for blue eyes (bb), then he will have blue eyes. But what if someone inherits two different genes? What if that person gets a big B from one parent and a little b from the other (Bb)? Well, that person will have brown eyes, because the gene for brown eyes is dominant, and it "wins."

Mother Bb (Brown Eyes)

	B	b
b	Offspring 1: Brown Eyes **Bb**	Offspring 2: Blue Eyes **bb**
b	Offspring 3: Brown Eyes **Bb**	Offspring 4: Blue Eyes **bb**

Father bb (Blue Eyes)

Recessive genes only "show" when there is a double recessive, such as bb, where the offspring got a little b from each parent. Therefore, traits from recessive genes, like blue eyes, only show up when both parents carry the gene. How does this relate to diseases of pets? Well, defective genes (genes for diseases) are commonly recessive. That means an animal has to have two defective genes, one from each parent, to develop the disease.

In the theoretical example below, the gene big K represents healthy kidneys and is a dominant gene, while the gene little k represents kidney disease and is recessive.

		Mother Kk (Healthy)	
		K	**k**
Father Kk (Healthy)	**K**	Offspring 1: Healthy **KK**	Offspring 2: Healthy **Kk**
	k	Offspring 3: Healthy **Kk**	Offspring 4: Diseased **kk**

If little k was a rare recessive gene for a particular type of kidney disease, it would be unlikely that two animals carrying the gene would meet and mate by random chance. But if an animal carrying the little k gene was mated to a related animal, it would be much more likely that this related animal also carried the gene, since they come from the same family and share genetic similarities.

Because most breeds were built on a small group of founding animals, they have a very limited gene pool. By breeding only within this group of related animals, who share common ancestors, the same genes are reproduced and amplified continuously. This is how it is possible for all members of the breed to have predictable characteristics, but also means that any recessive genes for genetic disorders lurking in the gene pool are likely to be matched up with each other because of mating between related animals. Many offspring will receive a recessive gene from each parent, and therefore will develop whatever inherited disorder is carried by that gene. (This is one reason why human societies have taboos against marrying a relative.)

Many pet insurance companies exclude these hereditary diseases from their coverage. The companies don't want everyone to have to pay a higher premium because some people have purebred pets that are prone to health problems. As a veterinarian, I find that most owners of purebred animals have no idea when they obtain their pet of the predictable health issues that occur in that breed. This is something that is well worth investigating when you are thinking about getting a new pet. Mixed-breed pets tend to be healthier (and thus less expensive to care for), and far less likely to have conditions that are excluded from insurance coverage. If you do have a purebred pet, particularly of a breed that is predisposed to costly health issues, you may want to select a company that does cover hereditary disorders.

Coverage on vacation or while traveling: If you plan to travel with your pet, be sure to check if coverage will continue while you are away. This may vary depending on where you and your pet go.

Is pet insurance worthwhile?

On the one hand, pet insurance is a gamble. You have no way to predict whether the amount you pay in premiums will be more or less in dollar amounts than the benefits you receive. If your pet becomes ill during the policy period, you will almost certainly benefit. If you maintain insurance for a number of years during which your pet is perfectly healthy, you may lose money overall. On the other hand, the main purpose of health insurance is to have a safety net: to avoid the terrible predicament in which your pet suddenly needs lifesaving care that you cannot afford to provide, or that will unacceptably affect your personal or family finances. If a pet insurance policy can prevent this dilemma from becoming a reality, it may be well worth it to you.

CareCredit

CareCredit (www.carecredit.com) is a program that allows pet owners to make monthly payments on veterinary bills (and certain other expenses as well). Similar to a credit card, you must apply for this service, and a variable amount of credit may be extended based on your financial picture. Once you have used your account to pay a bill, you are then responsible for monthly payments until that amount is paid off. You can reuse your account as long as you still have credit left over from previous expenses.

CareCredit is a good resource for an unexpected emergency *if* you will be able make your payments comfortably. For balances over a minimum amount that are paid off within a specified time period, you don't pay interest as long as monthly payments are kept up. Basically, the program provides a payment plan for pet owners who need some time to pay a bill. However, bear in mind that finance charges will occur if you cannot meet the monthly cost, and be careful not to put yourself into a position of unmanageable debt.

Not all veterinarians participate with CareCredit. If you would like to use this program for a pet's medical bills, check to see if the practice accepts it. You or another family member can apply online from home, or the veterinary hospital staff can help you apply while at their office. Be sure to carefully research all the details of the program, as the information provided here may not remain up-to-date.

Dedicated Savings Accounts

If you are someone who has the discipline to manage it, a savings account dedicated to your pet's medical expenses is an excellent idea. Many people can afford to put away a small amount each month, but would not be able to manage a sudden, large veterinary bill. By putting a specified amount into a savings account at your bank each month, you will build up a nest egg that you can use if your pet suddenly needs medical help. In the meantime, your money will be making interest, and it will be available to you if another crisis should arise. If your pet remains healthy until middle or old age, the amount you have on hand will have grown to even more than what you put in due to the interest that has accrued over the years.

Many employers are able to deposit a portion of an employee's paycheck directly into a designated bank account. If this is a possibility for you, figure out the amount that would be affordable for you, and make the necessary arrangements. That way, the process is relatively painless, and you don't have to worry about forgetting. I always remember those commercials that tell us how much could be done for the price of a cup of coffee a day. The same holds true for yourself and your pet: For a dollar a day, you could stash away thirty dollars a month; after five years of doing so in an account that pays some interest, you will have almost two thousand dollars available if needed. If you can afford to put more in each month (or some months), even better. If you put away the price of a daily cup of double-mocha half-decaf soy latte each month, you and your pet will be in great shape in no time!

THE BOTTOM LINE . . .

I know that nobody wants to think about a pet getting sick. Especially if you just got a brand-new kitten or puppy, it's the last thing on your mind. However, the reality is that your pet will need medical help at some point, and now is the time to start thinking about how you're going to manage it. Just as parents begin planning for college tuition the moment their baby is born, you should have a strategy for your pet's health care from the outset. Talk to your veterinarian; since she knows you and your pet personally, she may be able to offer helpful guidance. Whether you choose pet health insurance, a savings account, or another method that works for you, the key to being able to provide the care your pet needs is to plan ahead.

PET HEALTH INSURANCE COMPANY WEBSITES

- AKC Pet Healthcare: www.akcphp.com
- ASPCA: www.aspcapetinsurance.com
- Embrace Pet Insurance: www.embracepetinsurance.com
- Global Pet Insurance: www.globalpetinsurance.com
- Pets Best: www.petsbest.com
- PetCare: www.petcareinsurance.com
- Pethealth (Canada): www.pethealthinc.com
- Petshealth Care Plan: www.petshealthplan.com
- Petplan USA: www.gopetplan.com
- ShelterCare: www.sheltercare.com
- United Pet Care: www.unitedpetcare.com
- VPI Pet Insurance: www.petinsurance.com

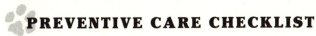

PREVENTIVE CARE CHECKLIST

To save money and protect your pet by avoiding preventable health problems, use this checklist as a guide. Your veterinarian may have other suggestions as well.

My pet is up-to-date on vaccinations according to his personalized vaccination program (see chapter 3).	☐
My pet has been spayed or neutered (ideally before first heat cycle in a female pet).	☐
My pet is on a monthly heartworm preventive.	☐
My pet receives flea prevention if appropriate for the season and area.	☐
My pet receives tick prevention if appropriate for the season and area.	☐
My pet is checked for ticks daily if appropriate for the season and area.	☐
My pet is protected from secondhand cigarette smoke.	☐
My pet receives regular home dental care.	☐
My pet receives periodic professional dental cleanings by the general veterinarian or a veterinary dentist.	☐
My pet receives annual veterinary examinations.	☐

PET HEALTH INSURANCE: WORKSHEET

Following are some of the factors to consider when choosing a pet insurance policy. You should be sure to understand all of these details before enrolling.

1. Does the policy provide coverage for preventive care? What kind of preventive care is covered? Examples include:

   - Vaccines.
   - Dental care.
   - Flea and tick preventives.
   - Spay/neuter.
   - Heartworm preventives.
   - Annual exams.

2. Will the benefits paid for the preventive care treatments your pet will need during the policy period outweigh the higher monthly premium for this coverage?

3. Does the company use set benefit schedules or pay a percentage of your bills?

4. How do the benefit schedules compare with veterinary costs in your area?

5. Is there an annual deductible, a per-visit deductible, or a per-incident deductible?

6. Is there an annual maximum paid by the policy? What is the amount?

7. Is there a maximum amount paid per incident or per system by the policy? What is the amount? How does the company define *per incident*?

8. Does the policy cover chronic conditions year-to-year, or will they be excluded as preexisting for the next policy period?

9. Does the policy cover hereditary disorders in purebred pets?

10. Are there restrictions on which veterinarian you can see?

11. Is there a multiple-pet discount?

12. Will your pet be covered during travel or vacations?

13. At what age are pets excluded from coverage?

14. What conditions are excluded from coverage? Ask your veterinarian about the likelihood of these conditions in your pet.

Epilogue

As I write these words, my cat Dov lies across the desk, purring contentedly. He loves to help me work and is willing to do whatever it takes: sitting just in front of the screen so I have to peer awkwardly around him, snuggling happily into my lap so that it's virtually impossible to type, or just staring at me in that dopey, adorable way that compels me to pause and give him a hug. Each of my pets has a unique role in the household (just as yours probably do), and we call Dov "the assistant"—if there's a task to be done, he's your cat. He's always right by my husband's side as Pete fixes a leaky pipe or installs a new appliance, and he has been my steadfast helper throughout the writing of this book.

Dov doesn't know how important his safety is to us, or how much we value his good health. He has no idea that the book he has so patiently co-authored is for him and all the other furry companions out there helping their humans through life. Our pets get us through the day (or the week, or the year): They greet us when we come home, they comfort us when we cry, they make sure we exercise, they entertain our kids . . . they have so many roles in our lives, especially just bestowing that living warmth that is so often lacking in modern life.

In turn, we are their guardians. Their well-being is in our hands, and our job is to protect them from harm and to do our best to keep them vital and comfortable as long as we can. It's a big responsibility. Our pets mean more to us all the time, and we have more options than ever before: in what to feed them, how to care for them, and how to keep them healthy. It's amazing that these choices exist; our pets are fortunate enough to live in a society where there is a grocery store aisle just for them, not to mention the advanced medical technology that is now available to them when needed.

I know that for a concerned pet owner, trying to keep up with the latest information can be a bit daunting. There has been a great deal of change in veterinary medicine over the last few decades, and these developments have occurred so rapidly that the profession itself hasn't had time to catch up or establish uniform standards. There is much diversity in the way veterinary medicine is being practiced, and this in turn has led to confusion among consumers who lack the facts they require to make informed decisions regarding their pets' health care. My goal has been to clear up some of that confusion, for you and others like you.

Hopefully, this book has provided a practical road map to modern veterinary medicine and given you the information that you need to feel secure in your ability to safeguard your pet's health. I want you to be a confident advocate for your pet and a proactive partner with your veterinarian. Don't hesitate to use the knowledge you have gained to procure the very best care for your animal companion. With someone like you on her side, your pet is one of the lucky ones.

Acknowledgments

There are many who deserve thanks. Truly, I am most grateful to the extraordinary animals who have touched my life, and to their "parents,"—my wonderful clients who so often have become dear friends as well.

A number of gifted veterinarians—too many to list here—helped with the book in a variety of ways, from practical advice to ongoing inspiration. A few of these include: criticalist Susan Hackner of the Animal Medical Center; cardiologist Don Schrope of Oradell Animal Hospital, and his wife, Katy, a veterinary internist who was my hero during my internship and residency; neurologist Deena Tiches of the Bush Veterinary Neurology Service; dentist Chuck Williams of the Animal Dental Clinic; dermatologist Jeanne Budgin of the Animal Specialty Center; Felicia Nutter of the Marine Mammal Center; and Marty Becker, who, in addition to being the author of numerous books, is an unfailingly kind and generous person. I cannot leave out my interns, past and present, who have made me proud and have always kept me on my toes. Thanks in particular to Cara Lane and Emmy Pointer, who took such wonderful photos of Fred the cat and more.

Support and suggestions from a myriad of friends, family, and colleagues have been invaluable. Many thanks to Gloria Archer and Holly Cate for their (constructive) criticism; Patrick O'Keefe and Anita Edson for being cheerleaders; Gil Shapiro for going out of his way (and being such a great dad to his cats); my father for his calm wisdom; and Michelle Falcon for knowing (almost) everything. I am deeply appreciative of the sharp legal minds of Chris Green and Laura Ireland-Moore, and of all they do to help animals; my gratitude also to David Wolfson for his thoughtful counsel.

Heartfelt thanks to the whole group at Cueball, including Tony Tjan for his boundless energy and persistence, and Elizabeth Xanthopoulos and Jill Kravetz for their insight and dedication. Evelyn Battaglia taught me so much—I hope I can remember it all. Sandra Macdermott's talent will help readers to visualize all that can be done for their pets. I am also grateful for the support of Nina Munk of urbanhound.com, Andy and Kate Spade, and especially Dr. Mehmet Oz, who has benefited the health of so many.

I am indebted to the ASPCA for giving me the best job ever and encouraging me to help make Bergh Memorial Animal Hospital the most amazing animal hospital in the world—which it is. Where else can animals from every walk of life be treated as equals, and receive the high-quality health care that each and every one deserves? Kudos to all the talented and compassionate veterinarians who work there, as well as the incredibly dedicated staff who want nothing more than to treat animals gently and make them well.

Last but far from least, endless thanks to Alexis Hurley—the eternal optimist—at Inkwell, and to all the folks at Ballantine Books: my editor, Christina Duffy, who is the soul of patience; Sarina Evan; Libby McGuire; Kim Hovey; Patricia Nicolescu; and Brian McLendon, whose belief made all the difference.

Bibliography

Abebe, W. 2002. Herbal medication: Potential for adverse interactions with analgesic drugs. *Journal of Clinical Pharmacy and Therapeutics* 27(6): 391–401.

Booth, Sarah L., Ines Golly, Jennifer M. Sacheck, Ronenn Roubenoff, Gerard E. Dallal, Koichiro Hamada, and Jeffrey B. Blumberg. 2004. Effect of vitamin E supplementation on vitamin K status in adults with normal coagulation status. *American Journal of Clinical Nutrition* 80(1): 143–148.

Cole, Morgan R., and C. W. Fetrow. 2003. Adulteration of dietary supplements. *American Journal of Health-System Pharmacy* 60: 1576–1580.

Corrigan, J. J. 1979. Coagulation problems relating to vitamin E. *American Journal of Pediatric Hematology/Oncology* 1: 169–173.

Cucherat, M., M. C. Haugh, M. Gooch, and J. P. Boissel. 2000. Evidence of clinical efficacy of homeopathy: A meta-analysis of clinical trials. *European Journal of Clinical Pharmacology* 56(1): 27–33.

Decaro, Nicola, Costantina Desario, Gabriella Elia, Viviana Mari, Maria Stella Lucente, Paolo Cordioli, Maria Loredana Colaianni, Vito Martella, and Canio Buonavoglia. 2007. Serological and molecular evidence that canine respiratory coronavirus is circulating in Italy. *Veterinary Microbiology* 121(3–4): 225–230.

Ellis, John A., Deborah M. Haines, Keith H. West, J. Hilty Burr, Arthur Dayton, Hugh G. G. Townsend, Edward W. Kanara, Carrie Konoby, Ann Crichlow, Karen Martin, and Garland Headrick. 2001. Effect of vaccination on experimental infection with *Bordetella bronchiseptica* in dogs. *Journal of the American Veterinary Medical Association* 218(3): 367–375.

Ernst, E. 2002. A systematic review of systematic reviews of homeopathy. *Journal of Clinical Pharmacology* 54: 577–582.

Ferguson, Ewan A., Janet D. Littlewood, Didier-Noël Carlotti, Rob Grover, and Tim Nuttall. 2006. Management of canine atopic dermatitis using the plant extract PYM00217: A randomized, double-blind, placebo-controlled clinical study. *Veterinary Dermatology* 17(4): 236–243.

Habacher, Gabriele, Max H. Pittler, and Edzard Ernst. 2006. Effectiveness of acupuncture in veterinary medicine: Systematic review. *Journal of Veterinary Internal Medicine* 20: 480–488.

Hagman, Ragnvi. 2004. New aspects of canine pyometra. Doctoral thesis, Swedish University of Agricultural Sciences.

Innes, J. F., C. J. Fuller, E. R. Grover, A. L. Kelly, and J. F. Burn. 2003. Randomized, double-blind, placebo-controlled parallel group study of P54FP for the treatment of dogs with osteoarthritis. *Veterinary Record* 152(15): 457–460.

Izzo, A. A. 2004. Drug interactions with St. John's wort (*Hypericum perforatum*): A review of the clinical evidence. *International Journal of Clinical Pharmacology and Therapeutics* 42(3): 139–148.

Jonas, Wayne B., Ted J. Kaptchuk, and Klaus Linde. 2003. A critical overview of homeopathy. *Annals of Internal Medicine* 138: 393–399.

Kapatkin, Amy S., Michael Tomasic, Jill Beech, Cheyney Meadows, Raymond C. Boston, Philipp D. Mayhew, Michelle Y. Powers, and Gail K. Smith. 2006. Effects of electrostimulated acupuncture on ground reaction forces and pain scores in dogs with chronic elbow joint arthritis. *Journal of the American Veterinary Medical Association* 228: 1350–1354.

Kass, Philip H., William L. Spangler, Mattie J. Hendrick, Lawrence D. McGill, D. Glenn Esplin, Sally Lester, Margaret Slater, E. Kathryn Meyer, Faith Boucher, Erika M. Peters, Glenna G. Gobar, Thurein Htoo, and Kendra Decile. 2003. Multicenter case-control study of risk factors associated with development of vaccine-associated sarcomas in cats. *Journal of the American Veterinary Medical Association* 223(9): 1283–1292.

Kaye, Alan D., I. Kucera, and R. Sabar. 2004. Perioperative anesthesia clinical considerations of alternative medicines. *Anesthesiology Clinics of North America* 22(1): 125–139.

Kleijnen, J., P. Knipschild, and G. ter Riet. 1991. Clinical trials of homeopathy. *British Medical Journal* 302(6772): 316–323.

Linde, K., N. Clausius, G. Ramirez, D. Melchart, F. Eitel, L. V. Hedges, and W. B. Jonas. 1997. Are the clinical effects of homeopathy placebo effects? A meta-analysis of placebo-controlled trials. *Lancet* 350(9081): 834–843.

Miller, Lucinda G. 1998. Selected clinical considerations focusing on known or potential drug–herb interactions. *Archives of Internal Medicine* 158: 2200–2211.

Moore, George E., and Lawrence T. Glickman. 2004. A perspective on vaccine guidelines and titer tests for dogs. *Journal of the American Veterinary Medical Association* 224(2): 200–203.

Moore, George E., Lynn F. Guptill, Michael P. Ward, Nita W. Glickman, Karen K. Faunt, Hugh B. Lewis, and Lawrence T. Glickman. 2005. Adverse events diagnosed within three days of vaccine administration in dogs. *Journal of the American Veterinary Medical Association* 227: 1102–1108.

Moore, George E., Andrea C. DeSantis-Kerr, Lynn F. Guptill, Nita W. Glickman, Hugh B. Lewis, and Lawrence T. Glickman. 2007. Adverse events after vaccine administration in cats: 2,560 cases (2002–2005). *Journal of the American Veterinary Medical Association* 231(1): 94–100.

Mouzin, Douglas E., Marianne J. Lorenzen, John D. Haworth, and Vickie L. King. 2004. Duration of serologic response to five viral antigens in dogs. *Journal of the American Veterinary Medical Association* 224(1): 55–60.

——. 2004. Duration of serologic response to three viral antigens in cats. *Journal of the American Veterinary Medical Association* 224(1): 61–66.

Nagle, Terry M., Sheila M. Torres, Kim L. Horne, Robert Grover, and Mike T. Stevens. 2001. A randomized, double-blind, placebo-controlled trial to investigate the efficacy and safety of a Chinese herbal product (P07P) for the treatment of canine atopic dermatitis. *Veterinary Dermatology* 12(5): 265–274.

Ooms, Tara G., Safdar A. Khan, and Charlotte Means. 2001. Suspected caffeine and ephedrine toxicosis resulting from ingestion of an herbal supplement containing guarana and ma huang in dogs: 47 cases (1997–1999). *Journal of the American Veterinary Medical Association* 218(2): 225–229.

Overly, Beth, Frances S. Shofer, Michael H. Goldschmidt, Dave Sherer, and Karin U. Sorenmo. 2005. Association between ovarihysterectomy and feline mammary carcinoma. *Journal of Veterinary Internal Medicine* 19: 560–563.

Scott, Danny W., William H. Miller, Jr., David A. Senter, Christopher P. Cook, J. Edward Kirker, and Shaun M. Cobb. 2002. Treatment of canine atopic dermatitis with a commercial homeopathic remedy: A single-blinded, placebo-controlled study. *Canadian Veterinary Journal* 43(8): 601–603.

Singh, Nalini, Pramil N. Singh, and Jerome M. Hershman. 2000. Effect of calcium carbonate on the absorption of levothyroxine. *Journal of the American Medical Association* 283: 2822–2825.

Tizard, Ian, and Yawei Ni. 1998. Use of serologic testing to assess immune status of companion animals. *Journal of the American Veterinary Medical Association* 213(1): 54–60.

Twark, Lisa, and W. Jean Dodds. 2000. Clinical use of serum parvovirus and distemper virus antibody titers for determining revaccination strategies in healthy dogs. *Journal of the American Veterinary Medical Association* 217(7): 1021–1024.

Index

ABOUT THE AUTHOR

LOUISE MURRAY, D.V.M., D.A.C.V.I.M., is the director of medicine at the ASPCA's Bergh Memorial Animal Hospital in New York City. A specialist in veterinary internal medicine, she has been honored with many awards, including the Martin A. and Beatrice R. Weiser Memorial Award for outstanding research and the Carola Warburg Rothschild Human Animal Bond Award, and has been elected into the Phi Zeta Honor Society of Veterinary Medicine. Dr. Murray has appeared on national and local television, including ABC's *Good Morning America* and *World News Tonight,* CNN's *Anderson Cooper 360* and *American Morning,* CBS's *The Early Show, Fox News Live,* and NBC's *Nightly News.* She has also appeared on national radio, including XM's *Oprah & Friends,* and in print publications, among them *USA Today* and *The New York Times.* She lives and works in New York City.